The Neuropathology of the Alimentary Tract

The Neuropathology of the Alimentary Tract

Barbara Smith

M.D.(Bristol), Ph.D.(London), F.R.C.S.
Senior Lecturer in Pathology, St Bartholomew's Hospital Medical College
Honorary Consultant Histopathologist, St Bartholomew's Hospital, London

Foreword by

Basil C. Morson

V.R.D., M.A., D.M., F.R.C.S., F.R.C. Path. Consultant Pathologist & Director of the Research Department, St Mark's Hospital, London; Honorary Senior Lecturer, Royal Postgraduate Medical School of London

Edward Arnold

First published 1972
by Edward Arnold (Publishers) Ltd.
25 Hill Street,
London WIX 8LL

ISBN: 0 7131 4196 4

Printed in Great Britain by
Butler & Tanner Ltd, Frome and London

Foreword

Histopathology is making an increasing contribution to progress in the diagnosis, treatment and pathogenesis of gastroenterological disorders. This book shows how the development of a special technique has opened up a new approach to the study of the neuromuscular mechanism of the gastrointestinal tract. Dr. Barbara Smith shows us in this scholarly work how she has used this technique in the study of surgical specimens and animal models of human disease to give information which is valuable to the surgeon and physician in clinical practice. This is the best kind of clinical pathology. There is also a comprehensive bibliography from which Dr. Smith has drawn upon the experience of others and integrated this with her own studies. This alone provides a valuable bank of knowledge for anyone wishing to investigate these diseases. This book shows that neuropathology has an important contribution to make to our knowledge of the motor function of the gastrointestinal tract. For the diagnostic histopathologist it shows up the limitations of conventional techniques and adds a new dimension to the interpretation of microscopic changes in the nerve fibres and ganglion cells of the gut wall. But for the gastroenterological surgeon, physician or radiologist interested in the investigation of gastrointestinal motility it should have an even wider appeal.

B. C. M.

Preface

Some of the material used in this work was given to me by Dr. Basil Morson, to whom I am also very grateful for much help and encouragement. The rest was sent to me by a number of surgeons and pathologists in many centres. These cases are not common, and unless one can collect material from a wide area, one cannot draw any useful conclusions, and I am very indebted to them for their trouble.

This study would not have been possible without the technical skill of Mr. Adrian Pirson, who made all the histological preparations. His ability to do consistently good and repeatable silver stains on material, some of which arrived in poor condition, made it possible to make firm statements, and even sometimes diagnoses, on nearly all the cases sent. I am also grateful to Mr. Peter Crocker for coping so well with the difficulties of photographing sections which are 100 μ thick, and in which the important features are all in different planes.

Contents

1 Introduction

If an individual is to enjoy normal health and comfort, the food he eats must be able to pass through the gastrointestinal tract without hindrance and at a reasonable speed. The bolus must pass from the oesophagus into the stomach with ease and reflux of gastric acid be prevented. It must remain in the stomach for some time, where it is kneaded by gastric contractions and exposed to gastric enzymes until it is reduced to a semi-liquid consistency. Only then is it allowed to pass into the duodenum. Transit times through the small intestine are very variable in man. They must, however, be long enough to ensure adequate absorption and short enough to get one meal out of the way before the next comes along. Much of the water and some electrolytes are absorbed in the colon. If the faeces remain too long in the colon they become very hard and this may result in secondary complications, such as anal fissure, haemorrhoids and possibly diverticular disease.

It is thus obviously important that the passage of food through the intestine should be adequately regulated. Queues in doctors' surgeries bear witness to the complaints which may arise when, for one reason or another, this regulation is faulty. The control of intestinal motility is by the autonomic nervous system consisting of the cerebral autonomic centres, the extrinsic sympathetic and parasympathetic systems and the intrinsic myenteric plexus.

The autonomic nervous system has been very little studied pathologically, and in man little enough is known even of the anatomy of the peripheral ganglia. It has therefore been necessary, in order to study these problems, to devise a technical method which shows the anatomy of the myenteric plexus adequately, and then to examine a range of normal material. Against this background it has been possible to make a new approach to the diseases of alimentary innervation and to describe the morbid histology. There are a number of diseases both congenital and acquired in which the myenteric plexus is absent or destroyed over a localised area of the gastrointestinal tract. They produce considerable ill-health and occasionally death, but little has been recorded of their pathology or pathogenesis.

The nerve cells of the myenteric plexus are outside the blood–brain barrier, and do not have the protection afforded to those of the neuraxis. They are therefore liable, together with the cells of the posterior root ganglia, to be damaged by circulating neurotoxic drugs. Peripheral and autonomic neuropathies are common side-effects of drugs, and doctors do not always consider, when the patient comes complaining of abdominal distension or constipation, that it is the result of the tranquillisers he has been giving him. In some instances of prolonged therapy the damage to the autonomic neurones becomes irreversible. In order to emphasise this point animal experiments were done to show the sort of damage which is produced by some common drugs.

A knowledge of the anatomy and pathology of any tissue must form the basis of good clinical medicine. Nearly all the conditions described here can be considerably improved or even cured by treatment. Many others could be prevented by a better understanding of drug action. Patients with abnormalities of gastrointestinal motility are not often in immediate danger of death, but their condition may make their life extremely uncomfortable. The misery is increased by the fact that they are frequently regarded as 'functional' by their friends and doctors. It is the object of this study to try to help the clinician to make the very difficult distinction between 'functional' and 'organic' disorders in this field, as well as to put some of the better known ones on a firmer pathological basis.

2 The myenteric plexus in animals

(a) Anatomy

Previous studies of the anatomy of the myenteric plexus have been done mainly in animals. There are a number of interspecies differences in the innervation of the alimentary canal as there are in the canal itself. The size of the animal and particularly the distance of the intestine from the vagal centres in the brain-stem may also necessitate anatomical differences. The main lay-out of the plexus is the same in all species. It lies between the inner and outer coats and consists of groups of neurones, interconnected by bundles of nerve fibres arranged in a rather variable geometric pattern. This constitutes the primary plexus, and from this a secondary and tertiary plexus of finer nerves arise to supply the smooth muscle. The myenteric plexus communicates with both the submucous, and where present, the subserous plexus.

In 1847, Remak, the first man to demonstrate the unmyelinated nerve fibre, described nerves to the gut running in the mesentery, and ending in the muscle coats. This was probably the earliest intimation that the gut had its own nerve supply. Ten years later, Meissner (1857) described ganglion cells and a plexus of nerves in the submucous coat of the intestine. It was, however, Auerbach who first made a complete description of the myenteric plexus. He was a Jew, and for most of his life was not allowed access to a laboratory. His main work was done at his own expense, in a room in his private house with very primitive tools. The original account of the plexus was published, not in a scientific journal, but as a pamphlet and sold for a few pence. In 1862 there appeared a tract entitled *Ueber einen plexus myentericus, einen bisher unbekannten ganglionervösen Apparat in Darmkanal der Wirbelthiere*. He used material from a number of species, including man, and described ganglion cells connected by unmyelinated nerve fibres, although neither this, nor a later publication (Auerbach, 1864), are illustrated. He knew that the plexus extended throughout the gastrointestinal tract, and that its function was to initiate peristaltic contractions. Dogiel (1899), using a methylene blue intra-vital technique, described three types of cells in the myenteric plexus. Type 1 cells were multipolar, with short branching dendrites and an axon. The dendrites anastomosed with processes of similar cells to form a network, and he suggested that the axons were motor to the muscle fibres. The type 2 cells had long dendrites ending in the mucosa and were probably sensory, and type 3 were similar to type 1 but the dendrites were longer and did not anastomose. Other authors, including Kölliker (1896), have considered that this division into three types was artificial. Kölliker thought that the neurones were all of one type and motor in function. Cajal (1909) recognised the first two types only but considered that they were both motor, and Müller (1911) held the same view. In 1927 Catherine Hill reported in a communication to the Royal Society her findings in an anatomical investigation of the plexus. She had devised her own modification of the Bielschowski silver impregnation technique, which gives a good picture of the plexus in many animals. She described it as consisting of groups of nerve cells connected by fibre bundles. There were two types of neurones which could readily be distinguished morphologically. One type was dark-staining with a somewhat elongated body and short dendrites. It had fine uniform axons and she considered that it would be associational rather than purely motor in character. The second was larger and only lightly argyrophilic. It had long dendrites and might be unipolar, bipolar or multipolar. The nerve endings around the ganglion cells were axonal endings of the intrinsic neurones with some contribution from the vagus in the case of type 2 neurones. In 1931 Irwin using the methylene blue technique, described a similar picture in the guinea-pig. He did a thorough survey of the alimentary tract, and showed that there were variations in the numbers of neurones and ganglia and in their lay-out. In the same year Lawrentjew (1931) also described different types of neurones predominating in different areas. He thought that type 1 neurones were the post-ganglionic neurones of the parasympathetic vagal and sacral systems and the type 2 neurones regulated movements of the digestive tract. Honjin (1951) divided the myenteric neurones of the mouse into argyrophil and argyrophobe. He thought the argyrophil cells were probably equivalent to Dogiel type 1. They were star-like, polygonal or spindle-shaped and of varying size. They had one or occasionally two axons and a number of dendrites, and the cell body contained a neurofibrillar network. The axons were initially thick and smooth but diminished in calibre as they mingled with the fibres of the plexus and terminated on argyrophobe cells of neighbouring ganglia. The dendrites terminated on argyrophobe cells of the same ganglion or on capillaries. The argyrophil cells were much fewer in numbers than the argyrophobe, few ganglia containing more than one and some none at all. The argyrophobe cells were spherical, elliptical or polygonal and contained a yellowish-brown neurofibrillar network.

(b) The variations in the plexus at different levels of the alimentary tract

The enumeration of neurones present at different levels in the gut must be presumed to be subject to a considerable amount of error, as the cells are related to muscle which is contractile and extensible. However Sauer and Rumble (1946) calculated that in the cat there were 5 million neurones in the myenteric plexus and two or three times this number in the submucous plexus, making a total of about 20 million. In contrast to this, this animal has only about 1 million neurones in its posterior root ganglia. Irwin (1931), in the guinea-pig, showed that in the upper part of the middle third of the oesophagus the ganglia were small and few in number. At the junction of the middle and lower thirds the numbers reached a maximum of 1370 neurones/cm^2 and decreased again towards the cardia. In the stomach there was some increase in size and numbers of neurones from the cardia to the pylorus, being 3500/cm^2 proximally and 20,000/cm^2 distally. In the middle third of the duodenum there were 10,000/cm^2 and the neurones lay at right angles to the long axis of the gut. In the small intestine the arrangement was uniform throughout with the neurones parallel to the long axis, and the numbers were about 7500/cm^2. In the caecum the ganglia were large, circular and fairly close together beneath the taeniae and much further apart between the taeniae. There were three times as many neurones, 12,000, beneath the taeniae as between them, 4500. In the large intestine the ganglia were compact and presented no polarity. Again there were more neurones, 19,000, beneath the taeniae than between them, 15,000. In the sigmoid colon the neurones were larger than elsewhere in the large intestine.

Lawrentjew (1931) found in the dog, that type 1 neurones were abundant in the oesophagus and rectum and there were comparatively few type 2 neurones. In the small and large intestine type 2 was commoner. Murakami (1934) found only type 2 neurones in the caecum of the same animal. In the mouse, Honjin *et al.* (1959) found a variable percentage of the neurones were argyrophil in different segments of the alimentary canal. In the stomach it was about 1%, in the duodenum 3%, in the jejunum 5%, in the ileum 6%, in the caecum 10%, and in the colon and rectum about 15%. Maslennikova (1962) counted the neurones/cm^2 along the mesenteric border of the rabbit intestine, and found smaller numbers than Irwin. There were 3500 in the duodenum, 2900 in the jejunum, 2500 in the ileum, 1760 in the caecum and 3375 in the colon.

These differences described in the number of neurones present at different levels are related to the importance of motility in that particular region. They are highest at the pylorus and in the colon, where control of propulsion is paramount, and lowest in the small intestine. The function of the taeniae in producing haustration is assisted by the fact that there are more neurones beneath them than between them.

(c) The relation of the extrinsic nerves to the plexus

In 1899 Dogiel suggested that the extrinsic nerves to the intestine ended around the myenteric neurones. Cajal (1909) did not distinguish between sympathetic and parasympathetic, but showed a drawing of a nerve leaving the neighbourhood of a blood vessel to break up around the intrinsic plexus. Later writers (Langley, 1922; Hill, 1927; Modern and Thienes, 1936) maintained that there was no communication between the sympathetic endings and the plexus, the former terminating directly on the muscle fibres. In 1942 Botar *et al.* suggested that the myenteric plexus received only sympathetic innervation.

Experiments in which the extrinsic fibres have been divided in the mesentery have not produced consistent results, but possibly some parasympathetic fibres were divided as well. Johnson (1925) found no change in the plexus when he divided the splanchnic nerves. Waddell (1929) divided the nerves accompanying the large mesenteric arteries in dogs. He found that the finer intercellular fibres were reduced, but the large axons of intrinsic neurones remained. Using the fluorescent histochemical method for demonstrating catecholamines, Jacobowitz (1965) showed complete loss of fluorescence in the stomach, duodenum, jejunum, ileum and proximal colon after coeliac ganglionectomy in the cat and the monkey. The descending colon was normal.

One of the problems of the vagal contribution to the plexus is that there seem to be too few vagal fibres below the diaphragm to supply all the abdominal viscera. It would appear that one vagal fibre must 'control' a considerable area of intestinal wall. Langley (1922) suggested that one vagal fibre must be a 'mother' to several groups of cells. Jabonero *et al.* (1951) thought that the preganglionic parasympathetic fibres were in contact only with Dogiel type 1 cells. Honjin (1951) divided the right and left vagus, separately and together in the mouse. After section of the right vagus he found degenerative changes in a few fibres in the mesenteric, myenteric and submucous bundles and in most of the fibres which ended on the argyrophobe cells in the myenteric and submucous ganglia. Most of the fibres supplying the muscle coats, the mucosa proper and the blood vessels were normal. After section of the left vagus, there were similar changes but the number of affected fibres was less. After section of both vagi the animals could only be kept alive for four days. There were only a small number of degenerate fibres in the mesenteric, myenteric and submucous nerve bundles, a number of fibres in the myenteric plexus were intact. He concluded that most of the nerves ending around the argyrophobe cells were from the vagi, mainly the right, the rest were processes of intrinsic argyrophil cells. Most of the nerves to the muscle coat and blood vessels were sympathetic. The results of sectioning the mesenteric nerves suggested that many vagal fibres travelled with the sympathetic.

Using the sheep, Morrison and Habel (1964) found that after vagotomy there were more degenerated endings associated with Dogiel type 1 than type 2. Schofield (1962) performed cervical vagotomy or division of the dorsal and ventral nerve roots from T6 to L4, either central or peripheral to the ganglia, in a number of different species. After bilateral cervical vagotomy in the rat, there was considerable fragmentation of large fibres in the nerve fasciculi in the adventitial plexus. The medium and small fibres had broken into a series of spherical and spindle-shaped structures. There

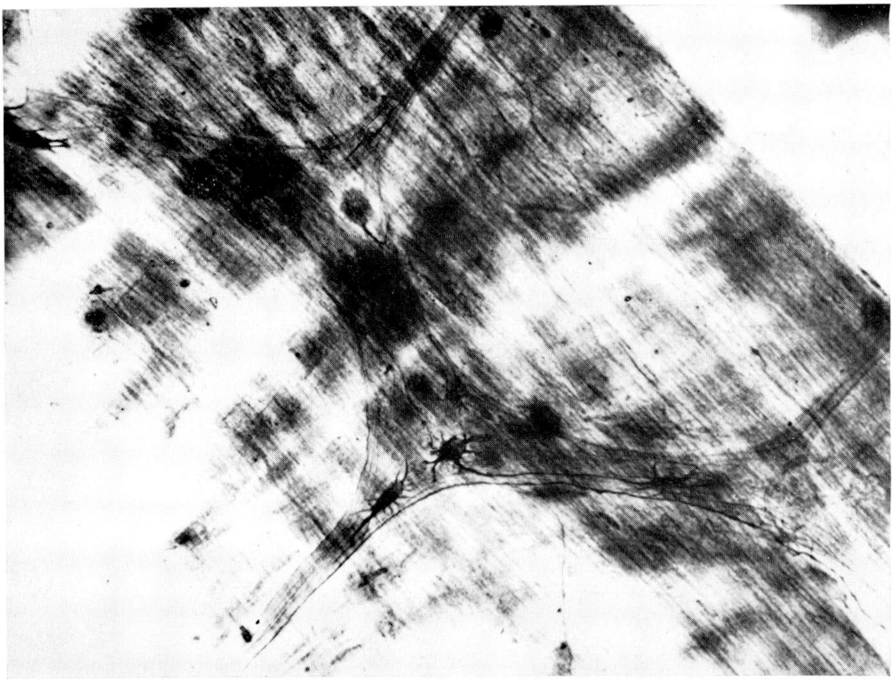

Fig. 2.1. The myenteric plexus of a normal mouse. This shows the morphology of the very scanty argyrophil cells present in these animals. It is very unusual to see more than one argyrophil cell in a ganglion and most have none at all.

were intraganglionic argyrophil swellings. After division of the spinal roots there was no definite lesion in the oesophagus. After cervical vagotomy the most significant change appeared to be an increase in the intraganglionic argyrophil swellings. Section of the spinal nerve roots showed similar findings to those produced by vagotomy. In neither case was there any reduction in the number of nerve fibres in the fasciculi. In the small intestine the changes were similar to those in the stomach, but less striking. After division of spinal roots T6 to L4, the changes in the large intestine were more striking than in the small. They consisted of a large number of intraganglionic argyrophil swellings and some loss of intraganglionic fibres. After division of the sacral nerve roots, there was little change in the histology. The changes produced in other species were similar.

The wall of the mouse colon is relatively thin, and the mucosa strips easily and completely. Whole mount preparations can thus be made of the muscle coats, including the myenteric plexus, and impregnated with silver. This has the advantage that only fibres which communicate with the submucous plexus are torn, thus reducing this type of artefact. With this type of preparation only a few argyrophil cells can be seen (Fig. 2.1). However the larger axons of both extrinsic and intrinsic nerves stain well and the lay-out is very adequately demonstrated. The sections can be 2 cm × 1 cm in size, which is quite a large proportion of mouse colon. On these sections the large parasympathetic nerves can be followed from the mesenteric border where they can readily be distinguished from the finer wavy sympathetic fibres. They are very few compared with the latter, sometimes running in the same bundle and sometimes separately as single fibres. When they reach the myenteric plexus, they divide at the first ganglion, two branches going to the next two ganglia and redividing, so that one parasympathetic fibre can obviously control a very large number

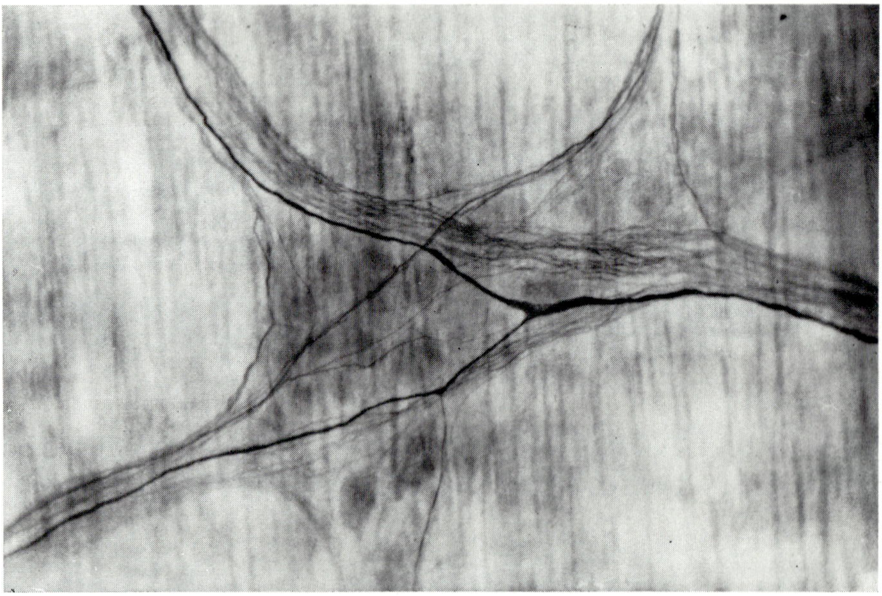

Fig. 2.2. The myenteric plexus of a normal mouse. The ganglion contains no argyrophil cells, but the outline of the argyrophobe cells can just be made out. The thick fibre is an extrinsic parasympathetic fibre which can be seen dividing to supply further ganglia, giving branches to the intrinsic neurones as it goes through. As many as 48 ganglia have been seen to be supplied by a single extrinsic fibre.

of intrinsic neurones (Fig. 2.2). Up to 48 supplied by one parasympathetic fibre were counted on one preparation, but this is an underestimate as fibres go off the section at both ends. The far more numerous sympathetic fibres enter the intestinal wall in bundles, which give off small branches to the myenteric plexus, in which they can be followed for only a short distance before being lost among the intrinsic fibres. The rest of the bundle goes direct to the muscle and through to the submucosa.

(d) The communication between the plexus and the smooth muscle

A constituent of the plexus which has produced more controversy than any other is the so-called 'interstitial cell'. These cells are smaller than the neurones and have processes running out at an angle communicating with each other. Kölliker (1896) considered that they were supporting cells and not neurones, as did Stöhr (1930). This was vigorously denied by La Villa (1897) and Cajal (1909). The former maintained that only neurofibrillar structures would take up methylene blue, and since these did so they were necessarily neurones. This is not strictly true, other structures will retain methylene blue, including reticulin and collagen. Cajal added observations on their argyrophilia to implement La Villa's statement. Lawrentjew (1925) thought they were a syncytium of strands containing neurofibrillae with no discrete cells. Hill (1927) described the interstitial cells as a network between the internal and external muscle coats, but did not commit herself as to their function. Boeke (1949) stated that these cells were similar to the primitive ganglion cells of invertebrates and were neuronal, a view shared by Li (1939). Spoerri (1949) described interstitial cells making direct contact with gastric epithelial cells, including the glandular and surface epithelium. Meyling (1953) was very definite that the interstitial cells represented the peripheral part of the autonomic system and that they were not schwann cells. Hillarp (1959), using methylene blue, said that they were neurilemmal, and they did not contain Nissl granules in sections stained for them. Richardson (1958) is the only author so far to have applied ultrastructural techniques to the problem, and in his opinion they were fibroblasts.

It does not seem necessary to postulate a secondary 'interstitial' cell network and there is no evidence for it on ultrastructural grounds. It is more probable that the connection between the nervous system and the muscle is by the autonomic ground plexus (Richardson, 1958; Hillarp, 1959). This consists of axonal ramifications embedded in schwann plasmodium which make contact with the muscle fibres. It is possible that adrenergic and cholinergic fibres are contained in the same schwann cell. There do not appear to be enough nerves to supply every fibre and some conduction is direct from one muscle fibre to the next.

(e) Histochemical studies of the myenteric plexus

The intrinsic innervation of the intestine is largely cholinergic, and it can be well demonstrated by the methods for cholinesterase (Plate I.1). (Koelle and Friedenwald, 1949; Koelle, 1955; Coupland and Holmes, 1957). The indoxyl method for esterase (Holt, 1959) although non-specific has the advantage that it is quicker, less inclined to diffuse, and it is easier

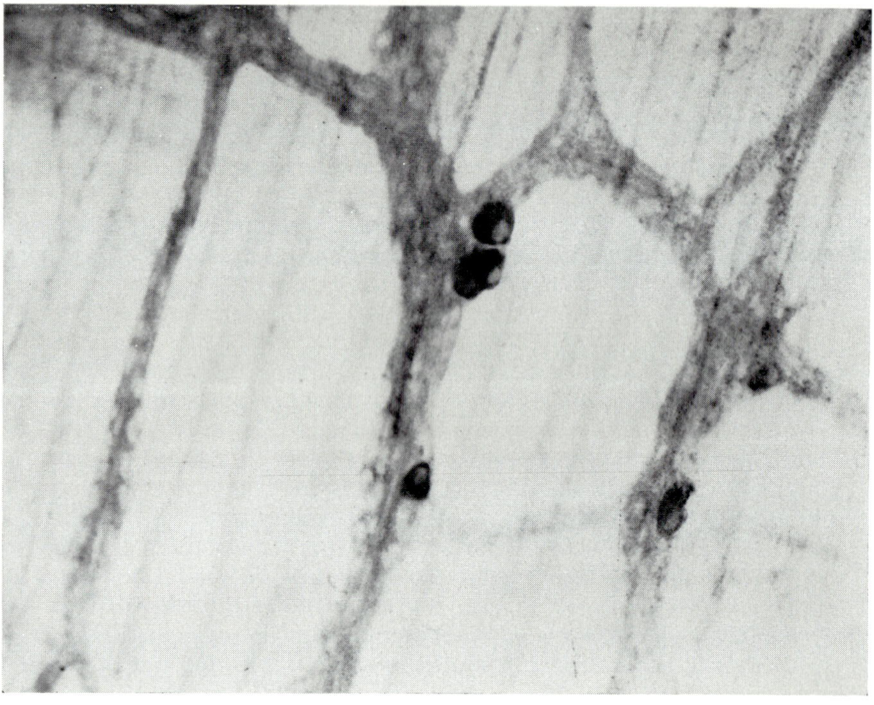

Fig. 2.3. Normal mouse. The myenteric plexus of a mouse incubated for acetyl cholinesterase for only a short time. Most of the cells are rather pale, but a few obviously contain much more activity than the rest. The significance of this is not known.

to counterstain the nuclei with neutral red. It gives a very clear picture of the plexus and the small amount of esterase, present mainly in blood vessels, does not spoil the section. In all types of esterase preparation the neurones and the nerve network are well shown. In acetyl cholinesterase preparations it is apparent that occasional neurones, not usually more than one or two in each ganglion, are more strongly positive than the rest (Fig. 2.3). Donhoffer (1959) has shown that a similar proportion of cells in the myenteric plexus were positive using butyryl thiocholine as

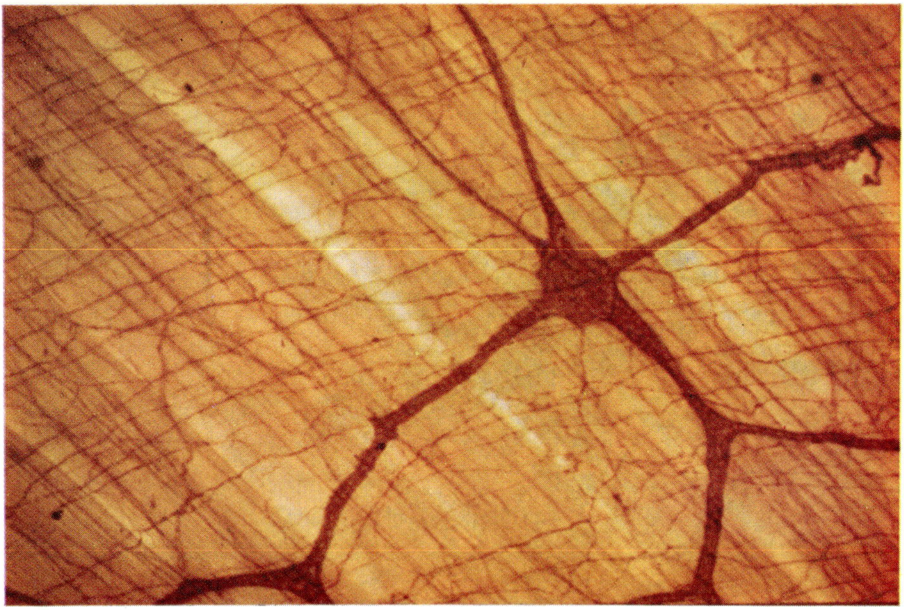

Plate I.1. The myenteric plexus of a normal mouse. A cholinesterase preparation of mouse colon, showing the neurones giving off branches to the smooth muscle. These neurones are argyrophobe and neither they nor their axons can be seen on a silver preparation. The axons of the argyrophil neurones remain in the plexus.

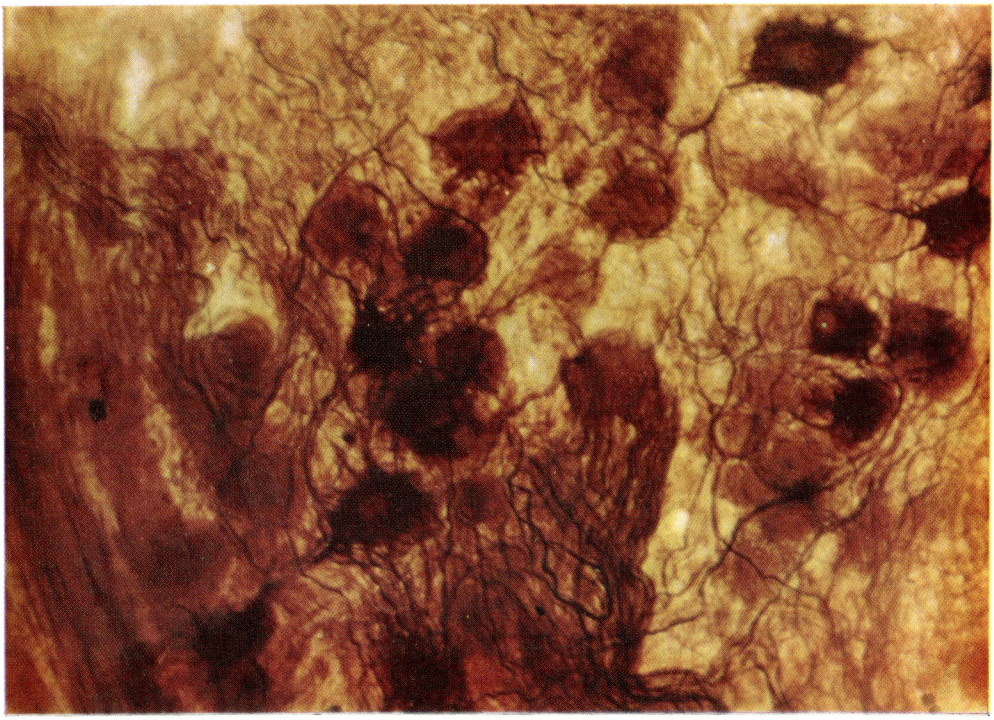

Plate I.2. The myenteric plexus of the normal human oesophagus. The ganglion contains argyrophil and argyrophobe cells. The neurones are more globular than those elsewhere in the gut.

[*facing page 10*]

substrate, suggesting that they also contained pseudo-cholinesterase. They could conceivably be the argyrophil cells. However it has not, so far, been possible to show that the silver-positive cells are the same as either those containing pseudo-cholinesterase or those with an increased content of acetyl cholinesterase, although the numbers are about the same. Leaming and Cauna (1961) in fact suggested that in the cat the argyrophil cells were cholinesterase negative.

Norberg (1964), using a fluorescent method for catecholamines, showed marked fluorescence in both the submucous and myenteric plexuses. Under high power this fluorescence appeared to surround the ganglion cells, but there were no adrenergic neurones. Jacobowitz (1965) in a similar investigation of the cat and the monkey found fluorescent fibres in the plexus and in the smooth muscle. After removal of the coeliac ganglion, all fluorescence was lost. Baumgarten (1967) could also find no fluorescent neurones in human colon. The catecholamine-containing fibres entered with the blood vessels and were distributed within the muscular layers and the ganglia of the submucous and myenteric plexus. In the stomach and small intestine there were only a few fibres in the muscle but the numbers increased towards the distal large intestine and there was a dense plexus around the sphincter ani.

Marks *et al.* (1962) used radioautographic localisation of tritiated noradrenaline in mice. They found it in the myenteric plexus but there was no uptake in nerve fibres or muscle layers. They suggested that the uptake and storage of noradrenaline was localised in the neural elements of the myenteric plexus.

In diagnostic practice, histochemical preparations are not as useful as might be anticipated. The cholinesterase-stained sections show the normal anatomy well, particularly in animals, but are of little value in pathological states except Hirschsprung's disease, and even there, there are simpler methods of getting the same information.

3 The myenteric plexus in man

(a) Method of examination

In order to examine the myenteric plexus in man it is necessary to cut sections in the plane of the plexus, that is, parallel to the intestinal wall. The specimen from the theatre or post-mortem room is washed through, ligatured at one end, distended with formalin under gravity, and ligatured at the other end. It is then completely immersed in a bath of formalin and left. If the specimen is small it may be necessary to suture rather than ligature the ends. This procedure puts the gut wall on the stretch and irons out the folds. An alternative procedure, if only a small amount of material is available, is to open it out and lay it flat on a piece of card, pressing it gently. After leaving it for 5 minutes to adhere to the card, it is put in a jar of formalin. It will not come off the card and the latter is sufficiently firm not to bend significantly when wet.

As in all silver preparations the duration of formalin fixation is important. This is because when tissue is placed in neutral 10% formalin or formal saline, the pH of the fluid gradually falls. Formalin fixes optimally at pH 7, but silver impregnation is more efficient at a somewhat lower pH. It is possible to lower the pH gradually with buffers, but this is time-consuming, and nature performs the task quite well if the formalin is not changed. The chemistry of the effect of formalin fixation in this context is not known, but it is very important. Unfixed material cannot be impregnated, and if alcohol is used as a fixative, special silver stains must be used. The mercury-containing fixatives do not give good results. Fixation should never be less than a week, and preferably longer. If the first impregnations are unsatisfactory, they can sometimes be improved by repeating them after a further fortnight's fixation.

After fixation the intestinal loop is opened and blocks about 2 cm × 1 cm taken at regular intervals along the material. A slice is taken from one end of each block for paraffin section. It is then placed mucosal surface down on the freezing module of a sledge-type microtome, and sections cut at 100 μ. The junction between the outer and inner muscle coats can be seen naked-eye, as the sections are cut. As the opened-out tube can never be quite flat, this will usually appear on two or three sections. They can then be stained by any of the double-impregnation silver methods which are used for peripheral nervous tissue. A method which is good, and reasonably quick, is that described by Schofield (1960). By cutting thinner sections, usually about 20–40 μ, it is possible to make good preparations with standard stains such as sudan black, periodic acid/Schiff and cresyl violet.

(b) Normal appearances

Paraffin sections of the intestine cut transversely, show a number of ganglion cells and schwann cells between the two muscle coats. Comparatively little information can be gained from this technique about the plexus itself, except whether or not it contains an inflammatory exudate. It does show the state of the mucosa, and the appearance and thickness of the muscle coats. Attempts have been made to interpret neuronal changes on paraffin sections and these have come in for very justifiable criticism (Rintoul and Kirkman, 1961). One of the main difficulties is that nervous tissue contains a lot of lipid, some of which is leached out in the processing. This leads to apparent shrinkage and vacuolation of neurones and may result in irregular staining which is artefactual. However in cases in which neuronal changes can be seen on silver preparations, the neurones in a haematoxylin and eosin stain are sometimes grossly triangulated and the cytoplasm stains a reddish purple. This may be significant of some pathology if only that of anoxia.

The appearances seen in the silver preparations from a normal adult which have been properly prepared are consistent. The plexus consists of a mesh of nerve fibres containing 20 or 30 axons of varying thickness. There are usually one or two very thick fibres, which are darkly staining and regular in calibre. These can be traced back and shown to be the axons of intrinsic neurones. The other fibres are finer and difficult to follow any distance. They are a mixture of extrinsic and intrinsic fibres. The neurones are aggregated in ganglia at the angles of the mesh. Only a small proportion of neurones in each ganglion are argyrophil, and this varies in different sites in the alimentary tract. It is very small in the small intestine but higher in the colon. The argyrophil cells are large and variable in shape. They are pyramidal, rounded or oval, the majority having several axons and a variable number of dendrites, but bipolar and occasionally unipolar cells are seen. The axons enter the plexus and join neighbouring ganglia. They can often be seen to bifurcate, by this means supplying a number of ganglia. Some axons pass through a ganglion giving off branches to its contained neurones and then going through to the next ganglion. Eventually they become too fine to follow. The dendrites appear to end around muscle of its nerve supply for any length of time, a procedure which might well damage membrane structure, altering ionic permeability, apart from other changes. One electron-microscopical observation on oesophageal muscle in achalasia of the cardia has been published (Cassella *et al.*, 1965*b*). The changes described there, of disorganisation of myofibrils and an increase in ribosomes, are similar to those known to occur in denervated skeletal muscle.

Alvarez (1949) quoted some observations by Biedermann on the slug. This creature has 3 paired ganglia supplying the 3 segments of the body. If the ganglion supplying the tail portion on one side is removed, this part contracts down into a tight knot. This suggests that the function of the nerve supply is to stop the muscle contracting. Smooth muscle is very sensitive to many different stimuli such as stretch, trauma, changes in ion concentration and many others. It could be that the function of the innervation is to damp down this effect, so that the muscle does not over-react to every minor environmental change.

In cases of acquired myenteric plexus damage the hypertrophy is usually associated with considerable dilatation of the gut. This, of course, makes the actual increase in muscle mass even more impressive. An important stimulus to smooth muscle contraction is stretch. If there is no coordinated peristalsis, the bolus is not moved on and the loop is continually being refilled from above, stretching the walls. This will increase the normal segmentation movements which are not under nervous control. Hyper-segmentation is a clinical feature of achalasia of the cardia, acquired damage to the myenteric plexus in the small bowel, and of the dilated segment in Hirschsprung's disease (Zuelzer and Wilson, 1948). This hyper-segmentation going on over many years could well result in a true work hypertrophy of these dimensions.

An interesting observation was made by Keeler *et al.* (1966). They gave intraperitoneal mepacrine to rats, a procedure which damages the myenteric neurones. They showed that the animals developed a thickened bowel wall in the space of 10–14 days, twice as great as that produced by rectal ligation. They also saw mitotic figures in smooth muscle cells suggesting that there was hyperplasia as well as hypertrophy.

Whatever the exact cause of the smooth muscle hypertrophy, and it may be a combination of factors, it is a constant feature of effective denervation. The thick bowel cannot, unfortunately, be diagnosed clinically, but at laparotomy it is a very helpful feature. It provides evidence of the cause of the obstruction and also the length of intestine which, if practicable, should be resected.

4 Changes seen in the myenteric plexus not due to primary disease

The difficulties in interpreting sections of this material are mainly due to inadequate preparation of the specimen. Distension of the intestine with formalin, by increasing the diameter, automatically makes the plexus flatter. If the diameter is small very little plexus will appear on each section. In addition, in the unstretched wall, the axons may appear concertina-ed and as a result show irregularities of calibre. This also occurs if the specimen is opened fresh and fixed flat, as there is then no tension on the wall.

Problems may arise as a result of inadequate staining. In a good preparation there should not be too much staining of the muscle nuclei, although there is usually a little. If this is excessive the procedure should be repeated as it tends to be associated with under-impregnation of axons. Reticulin may stain to some extent, but this does not matter as it is different morphologically to axonal material. Any given silver technique with a given thickness of section will stain axons only down to a certain calibre. Finer processes are not seen. In pathological material this is, in fact, an advantage, because one is really only interested in neurones and the primary plexus, and further detail could well serve to obscure this. However it is important that the technique should be consistent enough to show the same calibre fibres on all sections. It is probably not safe to report loss of axons without a corresponding increase in size and number of schwann cells.

Another factor which must be considered in surgical material is the technique and the time taken for removal. If the handling is long-sustained and rough, the neurones may appear very dark and the plexus may actually show some oedema. In post-mortem material, the mode of death is important, as prolonged ante-mortem anoxia may again produce dark and sometimes swollen neurones. Since many patients suffer a period of failing circulation and respiratory insufficiency before death, post-mortem material nearly always shows differences from surgical. Autolysis in post-mortem material makes stomach and small intestine unsuitable for this type of investigation, unless the autopsy is done very soon after death.

(b) Changes in the myenteric plexus due to neurological disease outside the gastrointestinal tract

Conditions in which the extrinsic nerve supply of the intestine is damaged may, under some circumstances, produce histological changes in the plexus. Babies born with a meningomyelocele have extensive abnormalities in the lumbo-sacral cord including the central neurones of the pelvic parasympathetic nerves. Examination of the colon in these infants dying in the first few days of life shows no changes from those seen in the normal neonate. However it must be remembered that the skeletal muscle of the legs may show little evidence of denervation at birth, although it develops later. It is possible that while the open neural plate is in contact with the amniotic fluid the neurones remain intact, and only degenerate after birth. A single case of an adult with a similar condition was also normal. This man of 30 had a flaccid paraplegia up to the level of L3 and was unable to empty his bladder. In spite of this, he had always had his bowels open normally without enemata. This suggests that there may be an anatomical separation of the centres for bowel and bladder control. If the colonic centre were deeper in the plate it might be less affected than that for the bladder.

Destruction or damage to the cauda equina in adult life produces a failure of colonic motility. Examination of such cases many years after the event, shows that there is very definite loss of plexus. Neurones are few and have presumably been lost from trans-synaptic degeneration and axons are very scanty. There may, in addition, be wavy bundles of fibres, which are not lying in the plexus and are obviously of extrinsic origin, This could be an attempt by nature to reinnervate an area from the nearest intact cells, possibly the lumbar sympathetic. It is doubtful if they have any function as they do not have adequate peripheral connections.

Extensive damage to the extrinsic innervation of the bowel can be produced by malignant tumours, particularly such conditions as retroperitoneal sarcoma. As with all malignant disease it is very difficult to assess accurately the extent of the anatomical lesion. However if the retroperitoneal involvement is pronounced the patients may develop postural hypotension. In these cases fragmentation of nerve fibres can be seen in the myenteric plexus, the axons of the intrinsic neurones remaining intact. Patients with spinal deposits or extradural tumour with malignant invasion of the posterior root ganglia also show some damage both to the extrinsic nerves and to an occasional fibre in the plexus. These fibres presumably either pass through, or have their cell stations in the root ganglia.

5 The oesophagus

(a) Anatomy

In man the oesophagus is a tube 24 cm long connecting the pharynx to the stomach. It starts at the cricopharyngeal sphincter and ends about 2 cm below the diaphragm. At about 2 cm above the diaphragm is the inferior oesophageal sphincter which is a physiological structure without any anatomical basis. Above this is the ampulla and below it, between it and the stomach, is the vestibule. This latter structure, which is a cavity 4–5 cm long, thus separates the body of the oesophagus from the constrictor cardiae, which also shows no anatomical thickening.

The gullet is lined by stratified squamous epithelium which is arranged in linear papillae. Underneath this epithelium is a thick layer of connective tissue separating it from the muscularis mucosae. At the gastro-oesophageal junction this is invaded by irregular masses of glandular tissue. The muscularis mucosae is very thick and is often broken up into bundles separated by collagen. The submucosa consists of loose connective tissue containing the oesophageal glands; there is no submucosal nervous plexus in this region.

In man the upper quarter of the oesophagus is striated muscle, the second quarter is usually partially striated and partly smooth, and the lower half is smooth. These levels are somewhat variable. The smooth muscle consists of an outer longitudinal coat and an inner transverse one. This inner coat is circular near its upper end, but it becomes more oblique further down, the posterior part being lower than the anterior. Lower down still it becomes a spiral. In the vestibule both coats are slightly thicker than above, but there is no sphincter. Between the two muscle coats is the intermuscular septum containing the myenteric plexus.

The nerve supply to the striated fibres at the upper end of the oesophagus arises in the nucleus ambiguus, travelling in the glossopharyngeal and vagus nerves. The neuromuscular communication is by motor end-plates as in skeletal muscle elsewhere. The extrinsic parasympathetic nerve supply to the smooth muscle comes from the dorsal nucleus of the vagus. The vagus nerve, at the level at which it leaves the ganglion nodosum, contains a large proportion of medullated fibres both thick and thin. However many of these medullated fibres leave the vagus with the laryngeal and pharyngeal nerves and the vagal trunk in the thorax is much less myelinated (Evans and Murray, 1954*a*). More medullated fibres leave with the nerves to the pulmonary plexus and as it enters the abdomen the vagus in the dog is almost unmyelinated (Chase and Ranson, 1914). As early as 1892 Edgeworth considered that the medullated fibres were sensory. Counts have been done in the cat by Agostini *et al.* (1957) who found 400 medullated fibres at the diaphragm out of 31,000 and they thought that these were probably afferent. In the abdominal vagus in the rabbit, Evans and Murray (1954a) found less than 75 medullated fibres out of 26,000. It is thus not true to say that all preganglionic fibres are myelinated.

The vagi pass posterior to the lung roots, incline anteriorly and medially, and divide into three or four branches. There is some variation of the method of branching as described by various authors (McCrea, 1924; Jackson, 1949; Mitchell, 1940; Rash and Thomas, 1962). The majority of cases seem to have a pattern similar to that described by McCrea (1924). Two branches from the left vagus pass to the anterior aspect of the oesophagus, and there unite with one branch from the right. These form a plexus on the anterior surface of the oesophagus, and from this one or two stems pass through the oesophageal opening to form the anterior vagal trunk. Branches from this supply the lower end of the oesophagus. The remaining divisions of both nerves pass to the posterior aspect of the oesophagus forming a plexus and from this a single posterior vagal trunk passes through the oesophageal opening of the diaphragm. The oesophagus is supplied by twigs arising from the stems as they are applied to the wall, and there is intercommunication between the two plexuses.

The sympathetic supply to the oesophagus comes from a number of different sources. The cardiac branches of the superior and middle cervical ganglia give twigs to the upper oesophagus. The neurones of the lateral cornua of the 4th to 6th thoracic segments give rise to axons which leave the cord with the motor roots and enter the corresponding sympathetic ganglia. From there branches are given to the oesophagus. Some innervation also comes from the greater splanchnic nerves as they pass through the thorax.

A striking histological feature of the oesophagus is the amount of the extrinsic innervation, particularly at the lower end. There are more sympathetic and parasympathetic nerves visible on sections taken in this region than anywhere else in the alimentary tract. Many of them are forming plexuses and possibly acting as connections with more distal areas. If this is so they would form a useful pathway if the main trunks were divided. There is free communication with the plexuses on the back and front of the stomach.

The myenteric plexus in the oesophagus is not arranged so regularly as it is in other parts of the gut. Most of it lies within the thick intermuscular septum, but it does encroach on both the inner and outer muscle coats. The geometric pattern of nerve trunks is not so apparent as it is elsewhere. The individual ganglia are large and the neurones they contain widely spaced. The nerve cells are globular or pyramidal with a large number of dendrites, and not as pleomorphic as in other areas (Plate 1.2, facing p. 10). The argyrophobe cells have a slightly brownish cytoplasm, whereas in the intestine they usually do not stain at all. They are thus much easier to see, but they do not have stainable processes. The proportion of neurones which are argyrophil is about 20–40%, higher than in the rest of the intestine. The nerve fibre bundles are thick and contain a large number of axons. They are wavy even in a properly prepared specimen and can be seen freely communicating with the extrinsic nerve bundles. The plexus is continuous through the gastro-oesophageal boundary.

(b) The physiology of gastro-oesophageal closure

There has been much discussion among physiologists as to the method of closure of the cardiac sphincter. It is generally agreed that there is no anatomical muscle thickening, although there is an area at the lower end, from 1–2 cm above the diaphragm to 1–2 cm below it, where the pressure is higher than in the gastric fundus. Lerche (1950) discussed the mechanism of the gastro-oesophageal segment. He said that as the larynx moved upwards during swallowing, the bolus entered the oesophagus and rapidly reached the ampulla. In this phase there was considerable elevation of the oesophagus and the inferior oesophageal sphincter could rise by as much as 1½ cm. The bolus halted briefly at the ampulla, the inferior oesophageal sphincter opened and it entered the vestibule. When the vestibule was full the inferior oesophageal sphincter closed, the constrictor cardiae opened and the contents were squirted into the stomach. After the expulsion the cardia projected into the stomach with eversion of the mucosa of the vestibule. The efficiency of the closing mechanism at the cardia is very considerable, and it is difficult to force the contents of the stomach back up through the oesophagus manually.

The normal function of the sphincter is, of course, not to hold up swallowed material but to prevent gastric reflux. It therefore does not have to resist the order of pressure which other sphincters do. In some animals which habitually hang upside down, such as the bat, there is a definite sphincter with thickening of the inner muscle coat (Fischer, 1909).

Botha (1962) suggested that the inferior oesophageal sphincter, when closed, leaves a small conical aperture. This is made water-tight by close apposition of mucosal folds. The folds close the cardia orifice flush with the surrounding gastric wall, so that pressure is evenly distributed. It will resist a fluid pressure of 100 mm of mercury, but will allow gas to escape.

The diaphragm is not part of the closing mechanism, but the latter can only work efficiently if the structures are in their normal anatomical position. The diaphragm is responsible for maintaining this. If it fails to do so and a hiatus hernia occurs, the sphincter will be incompetent and there will be gastric reflux.

6 Achalasia of the cardia

(a) Clinical picture

The condition of achalasia of the cardia has been known for a long time, and its treatment by intermittent dilatation preceded any knowledge of its mechanism by about 300 years. There is a much-quoted description of the condition by Thomas Willis in *Pharmaceutice Rationalis* (1672). He treated the patient by making a rod of whalebone with a button of sponge on the end and teaching him to swallow it. Initially the patient was near death from starvation but by this means he was maintained in good health for 15 years.

The disease is commonest in middle life, although cases have been described in the new-born (Thompson, 1950). There is no difference in the occurrence rate in the two sexes, but it is the commonest cause of dysphagia in women. Barrett (1953) has divided the symptoms into three phases. In phase 1 the patients are aware that there is something unusual about the act of swallowing. They sip their fluids because they cannot take a long draught. On radiological screening, the oesophagus between the arch of the aorta and the cardia is more active than normal. The bolus may be held up at the cardia for a few moments, but there is no permanent obstruction. It is noteworthy that even with only this degree of malfunction the act of deglutition is deranged. This phase may exist for months alternating with periods of normality.

In the second phase there is frank dysphagia with or without malnutrition. The patient notices that the oesophagus contracts and relaxes as food is taken. If too much is swallowed he feels distended and he may be aware that it has stuck in the oesophagus and has not reached the stomach. The feeling of distension bears no relation to the amount of food in the gullet and it may appear right at the beginning of a meal. There may be some substernal discomfort, but pain is not a prominent feature. There is regurgitation of material rather than vomiting and oesophageal contents may overflow on to the pillow or into the larynx at night. The condition is worse under stress and the patient frequently will not eat in company. He loses weight and may suffer from avitaminosis, but rarely dies from starvation. The onset of symptoms does not always correspond with the degree of obstruction and it is often impossible to know how long the oesophagus has been abnormal. Radiologically at this stage, the first mouthful may pass into the stomach if the gullet is empty. After this a hold-up develops in the lower inch, a little barium trickling through from time to time. The body of the oesophagus is hypotonic and dilated and normal peristaltic waves are absent. The only muscle activity in the lower oesophagus are tertiary waves which do not pass the food on, and sometimes even these are absent (Templeton, 1948).

In the third phase the oesophagus is so dilated that there may be mechanical obstruction between the sack and the neck due to kinking. The gullet is tortuous right up to the cricopharyngeal sphincter.

It is worth emphasising that in cases which have been followed radiologically, the deranged peristalsis of the oesophagus antedates the distal narrowing.

Treatment is by cardiomyotomy or dilatation.

(b) Physiological changes in achalasia

In achalasia according to Botha (1962) the oesophageal sphincter fails to relax following deglutition. There is no coordinated peristalsis, and there is a decrease in oesophageal tone with dilatation and hypertrophy. He said that the sphincter remained competent even after myotomy. Kramer *et al.* (1956) also described purposeless, non-propulsive contraction only. These authors and Botha showed that there was a normal or hypersensitive response to mecholyl and this occurred even in cases in which dilatation had not yet occurred. Creamer *et al.* (1957) said that the resting tone of the sphincter was not increased, but it failed to relax during deglutition. They thus confirmed the earlier observations of Sir Arthur Hurst (1934) who insisted that the condition was a failure to relax, an achalasia, and not cardiospasm. Kramer and Ingelfinger (1949) and Nemir and Hawthorne (1954) have also emphasised that the oesophagus is hypotonic and there is no muscle spasm. However as Rake (1927) suggested, it is possible that in the early stages of the disease before paralysis sets in there might be some over-stimulation of neurones and excessive muscular contraction.

(c) Pathology

Over the last thirty years evidence has been accumulating from pathologists and physiologists that achalasia of the cardia is associated with loss of myenteric neurones in the oesophagus. A number of workers have described cases in which loss or absence of ganglion cells in the plexus was found, including Rake, 1926, 1927; Hurst and Rake, 1930; Beattie, 1931; Lendrum, 1937; Kay, 1951; Cross, 1952; Trounce *et al.*, 1957; Adams *et al.*, 1961; Adams, 1964; Botar and Rubanyi, 1965; Misiewicz *et al.*, 1969.

Rake (1926) was fortunate to obtain material from an early case who had died from unrelated causes. The sections showed not only loss of myenteric neurones, but also a round cell infiltration of the ganglia. This was the first occasion in which plexus pathology had been described in this condition. Authors' reports have differed about the completeness and distribution of the neuronal loss, but it would appear that they are not always completely absent. Adams *et al.* (1960) have described some retention of neurones in the cardiac area and a complete loss proximally, with pharmacological evidence of an intact innervation at the cardia. Cassella *et al.* (1964) have also shown considerable retention of ganglion cells. If paraffin sections are used a very large number must be examined before any useful information can be obtained about the extent of neuronal survival. Using the technique described here it is possible to get the whole oesophagus on 24 blocks, usually 72 sections. This is not an impossible number to examine.

Cassella *et al.* (1964, 1965*a*, *b*) did electron microscopy on a number of cases, and found changes in the ultrastructure of the muscle. These consisted of detachment and displacement of myofibrils with ribosomes between them. These are similar to those seen in denervated skeletal muscle.

A somewhat different pathology was postulated by some previous workers. In 1902 Kraus described atrophy of the vagus in fusiform gullet dilatation and Heyrovsky (1913) and Loeper and Forestier (1921) also found a vagal lesion. Kimura (1929) in a more complete study found degeneration of neurones in the cerebral portion of the dorsal nucleus of the vagus, and in the caudal portion of the ventral with gliosis. A milder case showed a lesion only in the dorsal nucleus, the ventral being intact. The vagus nerve showed fragmentation. More recently Botar and Rubanyi (1965) reported pathology in the preganglionic fibres and Cassella *et al.* (1964, 1965*a*) showed Wallerian degeneration in the vagus. However Lendrum (1937) examined the vagus in 10 out of his 13 cases and found it consistently normal. Authors do not always give details of their histological techniques. Since apparently only a small part of the alimentary tract is involved, only a small number of vagal fibres will be affected and many of these will be unmyelinated, so that teasing osmium-stained preparations will not be helpful. With any type of silver-stained section the sampling error will be considerable and it may be difficult to see any pathology, as it sometimes is in motor neurone disease. It is noteworthy in this context, that not only do we know nothing about the state of the myenteric plexus in the stomach in this disease, but there appears to be little published information about the state of gastric motility or the gastric emptying time.

A condition, clinically identical with achalasia of the cardia, occurs in Chagas' disease associated with destruction of the myenteric plexus by the *Trypanosoma cruzi*. This disease is discussed further in Chapter 12.

Transient achalasia of the cardia has been described as a complication of vagotomy by several surgeons including Pierandozzi and Ritter (1966). Tanner (1964) noted that it was usually transitory and at worst could be relieved by a single dilatation. Dysphagia may also occur in brain-stem

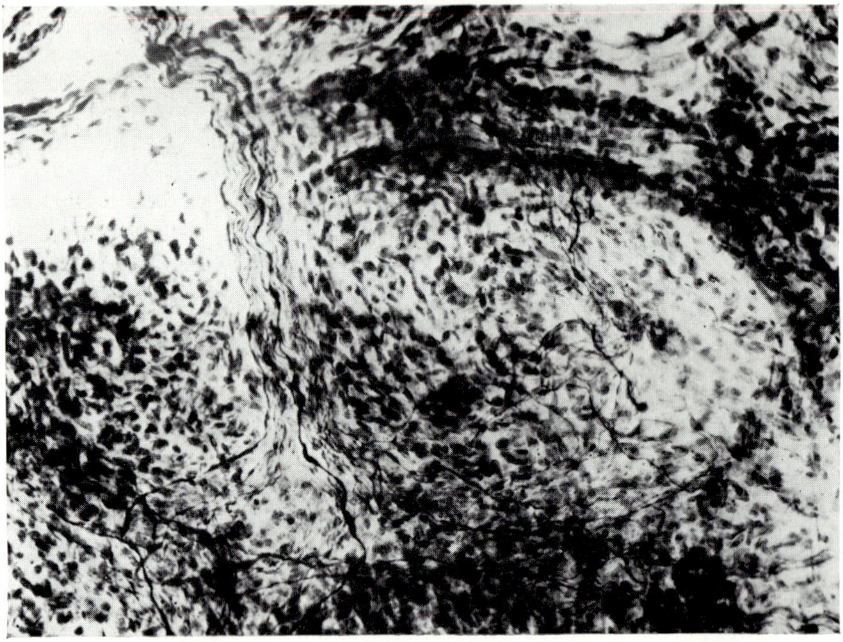

Fig. 6.1. The myenteric plexus in achalasia of the cardia. The ganglion contains no neurones and is replaced by schwann cells, fibrous tissue and a little argyrophil debris.

disorders such as motor neurone disease, anterior poliomyelitis, encephalitis and head injuries, but in most cases this is due to failure of the voluntary muscle in the upper oesophagus and pharynx.

(d) Case reports

The whole oesophagus of a woman who had died from an overspill infection was available for study. Paraffin sections showed no neurones, but there was no inflammatory reaction, the plexus being represented by fibrous tissue and schwann cells. There was severe hypertrophy of the wall, particularly the inner coat, and a modest amount of dilatation. The cause of this hypertrophy and dilatation is discussed elsewhere (Chapter 3. p. 16).

A large number of blocks were taken from the whole length of the oesophagus giving a very adequate sample of the wall, and no ganglion cells could be found. The ganglia were completely replaced by a mass of schwann cells with only occasional argyrophil debris (Fig. 6.1). Running among these schwann cells could be seen a network of varicose fibres, probably sympathetic, which appear to have been unaffected by the disease process in the ganglia. The extrinsic sympathetic fibres were normal. Some

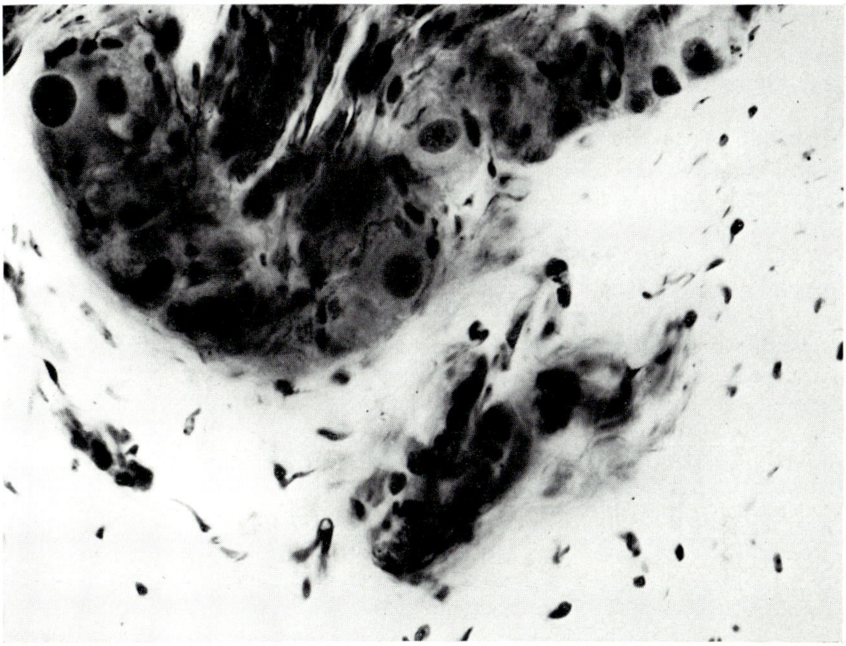

Fig. 6.2. The myenteric plexus in achalasia of the cardia. The argyrophil cells are lost but a few non-argyrophil neuronal nuclei can be seen. As it is the argyrophil cells which are involved in the gastro-oesophageal reflexes, the patient's symptoms are the same as if all the neurones are lost.

of the thicker fibres, almost certainly vagal, showed some fragmentation. The vagus itself, on the oesophageal wall, was examined by teasing osmium-stained fibres and by silver-stained sections. They showed no abnormality, but this does not exclude a lesion.

In addition to this post-mortem specimen seven biopsies taken during the course of cardiomyotomy were examined. These were not very satisfactory, because although the block was serially sectioned, only one or at the most two ganglia were visualised. In all but two cases these were replaced by schwann cells and contained no neurones. In the other two, argyrophobe cells were still present in fair numbers, but argyrophil cells were absent (Fig. 6.2). Provided that the residual neurones are argyrophobe they will not contribute to oesophageal reflex pathways and therefore the clinical effect will be the same as if all the neurones are lost. These argyrophobe neurones will, however, react as neurones to pharmacological stimulants.

(e) The experimental production of achalasia in animals

A number of attempts have been made to inhibit or destroy the myenteric neurones experimentally. Alnor (1958) produced cold lesions by applying CO_2 snow to the cardia in rabbits and dogs. Deloyers *et al.* (1959) used infiltration of the oesophageal wall with phenol in cats. They claimed that it produced specific damage to the neurones and consequent achalasia. Thomas and Trounce (1960) gave atropine and hexamethonium to guinea-pigs. They showed that while the drugs were active there was delay in the passage of food into the stomach and no coordinated peristalsis. Koelle and Gilman (1946) gave di-isopropyl-fluorophosphate (DFP) to several species of mammal three times weekly for a varying number of weeks and showed that they developed dysphagia. In one dog there was probably some degeneration of the neurones. This same type of experiment was repeated in dogs by Harris *et al.* (1960). They found that the animals developed oesophageal aperistalsis with failure of relaxation of the oesophageal sphincter. The oesophagus did not contract when distended by a balloon. Okamoto, Iwasaki, Veda and Takeda (1964) used the technique devised by Hukuhara (1961). They injected tyrode solution, together with a small amount of corrosive sublimate, into the oesophageal arteries for one hour. The dogs developed achalasia with hypertrophy of the smooth muscle. There was loss of neurones, the ganglia being full of supporting cells and the extrinsic nerves were normal. Earlam *et al.* (1967) using a similar method produced neuronal damage and fall-out in the dog's oesophagus but there was only a temporary change in motility. The surviving animals recovered clinically.

In addition to myenteric plexus damage, achalasia can be produced in animals by vagal lesions, although in most cases the condition is only transient. In 1906 Meltzer and Auer stimulated the peripheral end of the cut vagus and produced a tetanic contraction of the whole oesophagus. If they stimulated the central end only the upper part of the oesophagus contracted and sometimes there was relaxation of the cardia. Carlson and Luckhardt (1921) used turtles, and after vagal section they found hypertonus of the circular muscle of the oesophagus and cardia. If they stimulated the vagus, they found the reverse. Carlson *et al.* (1922*a*, *b*) sectioned vagi in the cat. They could produce cardiospasm for 3 to 15 minutes, sometimes longer. They suggested that the vagus contained motor and inhibitory nerves. If the tone in the oesophagus was high at the time of stimulation it produced inhibition, if it was low, contraction. Knight (1934) found, also in the cat, that bilateral vagotomy paralysed and dilated the oesophagus and contracted the sphincter. Grondahl and Haney (1940) produced achalasia by vagal section in the thorax and circumferential incision of the oesophagus down to the mucosa. Vagotomy alone in their hands was not effective. They suggested that the fibres which control relaxation of the cardia run down in the wall of the oesophagus. Lehmann (1945) also showed that reflex relaxation of the cardia, in response to distension of the body of the oesophagus, was abolished by transection of the wall, but this would also divide the vagus. Long *et al.* (1958) did a high cervical vagotomy in a number of dogs and observed dysphagia and the absence of peristaltic waves. Carveth *et al.* (1960) had a similar result with bilateral hilar vagotomy. The animals regurgitated undigested food. There was a dilated lower oesophagus and some retention of contrast medium after deglutition. The last four groups of workers all used the dog for their experiments. This animal has striated muscle throughout the oesophagus and a circular band of smooth muscle at the lower end acting as a sphincter (Mann and Shorter, 1964). It thus differs considerably in anatomy and mechanism from man.

A particularly interesting experiment was done by Higgs *et al.* (1965). They produced electrolytic lesions in the brain-stem in cats and dogs. They found that in the former, lesions of the dorsal vagal nucleus produced a reduction of relaxation in the gastro-oesophageal sphincter, and in the latter only lesions in the nucleus ambiguus. They suggest that this is related to the fact that in the cat oesophagus there is smooth muscle which is controlled by the dorsal vagal nucleus, whereas in the dog the oesophagus is almost entirely striated and would be supplied by the nucleus ambiguus.

The cat would appear to be the animal with an oesophageal structure most similar to that of man, and experiments on this species are therefore more relevant than others. In these animals vagal lesions produce at least a transient achalasia.

(f) Pharmacology

Studies have been made of the reactions of strips of oesophagus removed at cardiomyotomy, particularly by Trounce and his colleagues. Trounce *et al.* (1957) took their strips from the constricted area only. They found that the muscle responded to acetylcholine and that this reaction was increased by eserine, blocked by atropine but not by acetylcholine. Five out of six cases responded to nicotine after eserinisation showing that there were ganglion cells present. In a further study (Ellis, Kauntze and Trounce, 1960) the dilated part of the oesophagus was investigated. In this case there was no response to nicotine, so presumably there were no neurones.

In a study of normal oesophagus (Ellis, Krauntze and Trounce, 1960) the response to acetylcholine was always motor and it never showed relaxation. The circular muscle of the cardia responded to electrical stimulation by relaxation. Adams *et al.* (1960) reported a reduction of cholinesterase activity in the dilated part of the oesophagus in achalasia, but this was much less marked at the cardia. Misiewicz *et al.* (1969) have done similar investigations on the distal 4 cm of the oesophagus in control patients and achalasics. The control strips of circular muscle relaxed in response to nicotine and DMPP (dimethylphenylpipirazine) but noradrenaline and isoprenaline produced relaxation blocked by pronethalol. The longitudinal muscle was relatively unresponsive and gave variable results with all drugs. These authors concluded that the relaxation of the cardiac sphincter is under beta-adrenergic control and in achalasia this control was lost.

As mentioned earlier the results of pharmacological investigation of isolated muscle strips may be altered by the fact that a variable number of non-argyrophil neurones may remain in achalasia, and these will more commonly adhere to the longitudinal coat. If they do they will respond as neurones pharmacologically and the muscle will not, in fact, behave as if it were completely denervated. The number of neurones remaining varies from case to case, and in some instances there are none at all. This might account for slight differences between one case and another. However these pharmacological findings broadly corroborate the histological ones, that the lower oesophagus is denervated.

There is some clinical and pharmacological as well as pathological evidence that the vagus may be involved in achalasia. The Hollander test is an indicator of intact vagal activity and is usually used to show the completeness of surgical vagotomy. Insulin hypoglycaemia is used to produce gastric hypersecretion and the amount of acid produced is measured. The motor limb of this reflex arc runs in the vagus nerve. Iordanskaya (1962) found abnormal Hollander tests in 6 out of 13 patients with achalasia. Woolam *et al.* (1967) did the same procedure in 32 achalasics and 8 controls. The controls and 18 achalasics gave normal results, 6 achalasics gave a delayed response, and 8 no response at all. It would thus seem that just under half the patients with achalasia have impaired vagal function.

(g) Aetiology

Achalasia of the cardia is a disease of adult life, and there is no evidence that the loss of neurones is congenital. The few cases which have been reported in infancy may have a different aetiology and in some instances have been associated with other conditions such as pyloric stenosis (Blades *et al.*, 1957).

The neuronal destruction could be due to a number of different causes but there are points in favour of one or two in particular. There are a few cases in the literature (Hurst and Rake, 1930; Cassella *et al.*, 1964; Misiewicz *et al.*, 1969) in which the ganglia have been full of lymphocytes. This would suggest an infective process or an auto-immune one. One would expect antineural antibody to produce a more generalised effect on intestinal neurones unless there is a chemical difference between those in the oesophagus and those elsewhere. Neurotoxins also tend to produce less localised damage unless there is a pharmacological reason why they should be concentrated at a particular site. Since the only cause of infective myenteric plexus damage which is known is due to a protozoon, the *Trypanosoma cruzi*, it is necessary to consider the common protozoal infection in this country, which is that of *Toxoplasma gondii*. This organism elsewhere produces a rather florid inflammatory reaction and antibody estimations have not so far proved helpful. However in an old case of Chagas' disease there may not only be no leishmania but very little inflammatory reaction left. The majority of cases of achalasia which have been studied pathologically have been of long standing and one is only able to examine what are, in effect, scars.

The most important question which must be answered before the problem of aetiology can be solved, is whether or not there is always a lesion of the vagus and brain-stem. In many reported cases, it is not mentioned and it is not known whether it was normal or whether it was not looked at. As has been discussed previously, however carefully the nerve is examined, it is difficult to be dogmatic about the absence of any lesion, so that only positive findings are valid. If there is a lesion, and particularly if there is also loss of neurones in the dorsal nucleus of the vagus, it becomes a disorder affecting primary and secondary neurones.

Cassella *et al.* (1964) have suggested that the lesion in the brain-stem is primary and that the loss of myenteric neurones is trans-synaptic. After lesions of the sacral nerves there is some fall-out of ganglion cells in the colonic wall, but it is nothing like as severe as that usually seen in achalasia. Involvement of primary and secondary neurones recalls other system degenerations such as motor-neurone disease. These are, however, always progressive and therefore every patient should eventually have an enormously dilated oesophagus. This is not so as some of them appear to arrest. Another possibility which is compatible with a lesion in the vagus is infection with a neurotropic virus travelling down the axons. These viruses are very eclectic, often only affecting one group of neurones. The fact that some writers have reported lymphocytes in the plexus might favour this hypothesis. Many years ago C. P. Symonds (1930) suggested that as the myenteric ganglia were homologous with the posterior root ganglia they might be subject to the same diseases. A localised infection with herpes zoster virus could produce this type of histological change both in the recent and the burnt-out phase.

The differential diagnosis between an infective and a degenerative aetiology might be resolved by establishing whether or not the disease is progressive clinically. Virus infections usually produce maximum damage at first onset and then the virus disappears, as in anterior poliomyelitis and herpes zoster, whereas a system disorder would pick out neurones one by one. Patients with achalasia of the cardia do get progressively worse, but the muscular incoordination can be demonstrated at a very early stage. The increase in symptoms could be due to an increase in thickness and diameter of the oesophagus.

In conclusion the symptoms of achalasia are due to loss of the reflex pathway through which the gastro-oesophageal segment is made to relax in response to the presence of a bolus in the ampulla. This pathway probably runs in the argyrophil myenteric plexus. The thickening and dilatation of the oesophagus is secondary to the denervation and increases the clinical symptoms.

7 The stomach

(a) Anatomy

The stomach varies considerably in size and shape in different individuals, and from time to time in the same individual. From the cardiac orifice two borders, the greater and lesser curves, separate the anterior and posterior surfaces, the cardiac incisura dividing the cardia from the greater curve, which passes up at an angle to form the upper border of the fundus. On the lesser curve the pyloric antrum is separated from the body of the stomach by the incisura angularis.

The gastric mucous membrane commences just above the anatomical cardia along an irregular margin known as the 'Z' line. The mucosa is thrown into folds or rugae which partially iron out as the stomach is distended, and along the lesser curve the rugae are parallel to the line of the stomach. The epithelium is columnar and arranged along tubular glands. The cardiac glands around the cardiac orifice are coiled and mucus-producing, but the fundic glands are straight, simply branched tubules, with a lumen which almost reaches the muscularis mucosae. In this region the glands contain mucoid cells, zymogen cells and parietal cells. The pyloric glands are shorter and less densely packed, and their branching is more complicated. The epithelial cells here are uniform and mucous in type.

The muscularis mucosae is applied almost directly to the base of the glands. The submucous connective tissue is not as loose as in the oesophagus but it does contain a submucous plexus of neurones.

The musculature of the gastric wall is arranged in three layers and not two as elsewhere, only the middle coat surrounding the organ completely. The three muscle coats are interconnected by muscle bundles. The outer longitudinal coat is continuous with the longitudinal muscle coat of the oesophagus, which divides into two bands, the larger band following the lesser curve and the smaller spreading out over the greater curve towards the pylorus. The centre of the anterior and posterior surfaces are thus devoid of the outer muscle coat. At the pylorus both bands converge to form a uniform layer which is to a large extent continuous with the longitudinal coat of the duodenum. The middle circular coat begins at the cardia as a continuation of the outer fibres of the circular oesophageal muscle. It forms a continuous coat right up to the pylorus where it constitutes the pyloric sphincter. The inner oblique layer is continuous at the cardia with the deep circular layer of the oesophagus. It fans out over the anterior and posterior surfaces without reaching either lesser or greater curves and gradually disappears. The pyloric sphincter is formed from a thickening of the circular muscle coat but it is not continuous with the inner coat of the duodenum, being separated from it by a fibrous septum.

At the cardia the intermuscular septum between longitudinal and circular muscle is initially thick but thins out quickly in the stomach. The line of the myenteric plexus is somewhat irregular, particularly distally, many ganglia lying among the bundles of the circular muscle coat, both in the stomach proper and in the pyloric sphincter. The network is not geometrical as in the small intestine, but the ganglia are connected by nerve bundles producing a random pattern. The ganglia are widely spaced, but the organ is so distensible it is very difficult to get any idea of the neuronal population, the number seen on a section depending on the chance size of the stomach at operation or autopsy. At the fundus the neurones are small and predominantly argyrophobe, many ganglia containing no argyrophil cells. Progressing towards the pylorus the number of neurones and their argyrophilia increases, and at the sphincter the proportion of argyrophil cells is quite high. The plexus is continuous across the pylorus into the duodenum.

The sympathetic extrinsic nerve supply to the stomach is derived from the lateral horns of segments D6–D10. They pass via the rami communicantes to the sympathetic trunks and then in the greater splanchnic nerves to the coeliac ganglion. Fibres from the coeliac plexus travel with the inferior phrenic artery to the stomach supplying cardia and fundus, other fibres running with the left gastric artery innervate the cardia, the lesser curve and both surfaces of the stomach to the pyloric antrum. Some branches going to the porta hepatis are situated between the layers of the lesser omentum. Fibres from the hepatic artery plexus are continued along the gastro-epiploic arteries to supply the region of the greater curve and the two adjacent surfaces.

The parasympathetic supply to the stomach comes from the dorsal vagal nuclei via both vagal trunks. The anterior vagal trunk breaks up into five or six branches, one group lying on the right and anterior, and the other on the left and deeper. The left group usually but not always forms a plexus. It associates with the plexus around the left gastric artery and supplies the anterior surface of the cardia, the fundus and the proximal part of the body of the stomach. The right group gives three branches, one to the lesser omentum and porta hepatis which may give twigs to the pylorus and the first part of the duodenum, one passes down between the layers of the lesser omentum parallel to the lesser curve and is distributed to the anterior surface of the pyloric antrum and the body of the stomach but does not reach the pylorus, and one follows the lesser omentum to the incisura angularis. The anterior vagal trunk communicates with the coeliac plexus along the left gastric artery. The posterior vagal trunk usually divides into two. The larger branch goes to the coeliac ganglion communicating with the other abdominal plexuses and the smaller supplies the posterior surface of the body of the stomach and the pyloric antrum.

(b) Physiology

In 1886 Hofmeister and Schutz examined the motility of the excised dog's stomach. They saw waves starting in the fundus and travelling towards the pyloric antrum. This contraction ended at the beginning of the antrum, thus dividing the stomach into two chambers. The entire pyloric antrum then contracted simultaneously, and finally the pyloric sphincter. In 1898 Cannon used x-rays to observe unanaesthetised cats and saw peristaltic waves progressing all the way to the pylorus. In 1911 the same worker, using the dog, described the movements of the stomach as tonic contraction of the cardiac portion with peristaltic waves running over the pyloric end. There was no fore-running inhibition. If the muscle was tonic, distension was a stimulus to contraction, at other times the wall stretched passively. In contrast to the rest of the intestine the peristaltic movements were not abolished by nicotine and if the myenteric plexus was divided by multiple incisions, peristalsis continued with only slight hold-up. Thomas and Kuntz (1926) confirmed that rhythmic gastric movements persisted after nicotine. They considered that the enteric nervous system brought about variations in the tonus of the musculature, and the amplitude and force of contraction. It initiated and coordinated peristaltic and other reflex movements in response to local stimuli.

Thomas (1957) reviewed the information which was then available about gastric emptying, some of which was obtained from pressure recordings with intraluminal balloons. In a cavity as large as the stomach the evidence obtained by this means may not always be reliable (Brody *et al.*, 1940). During interdigestive periods there are mild rhythmic pressure waves at about 3 per minute. These gradually increase in intensity until there are spikes of about 30 seconds' duration at progressively closer intervals. These are assumed to pass from the cardia to the pylorus. After prolonged fasting a state of sustained tonus or gastric tetanus may follow. When food is ingested contractions stop and relaxation occurs in front of the bolus. The stomach enlarges to form a reservoir, the intragastric pressure remaining constant. Minutes after the food is swallowed indentations occur in the region of the incisura angularis, deepening towards the pylorus. These gradually come to start more proximally and become more vigorous. The pylorus opens only intermittently, most material being forced back to the fundus.

8 Hypertrophic pyloric stenosis

Hypertrophic pyloric stenosis is commonly seen in infancy, although a similar condition has been described in adults. It is often called congenital but, in fact, in contrast to Hirschsprung's disease, symptoms do not start from birth, but usually when the child is a few weeks old. The incidence is about 3 per 1000 live births, 1 per 200 males and 1 per 1000 females (Carter, 1961). Wood and Smellie (1951) found that 51% were first-born as against 39% of the general population. There appears to be some evidence of a familial factor. Burmeister and Hamilton (1964) described a family in which the disease occurred in 4 siblings. Metrakos (1953) found 12 pairs of identical twins, both of whom had the disease and another 6 in which only one did. In a larger study, MacMahon and McKeown (1955) found 87 affected cases in 81 pairs of twins among 3982 children with hypertrophic pyloric stenosis. The incidence in twins was only slightly higher than in siblings. Carter (1961) found that 50% of monozygous co-twins were affected. He traced 174 male and 48 female patients who had at least one child. The sons and daughters were slightly more likely to be affected than siblings. Woo-Ming (1961) described a patient with the adult type of pyloric stenosis, whose male child had to have a Ramstedt operation. Fenwick (1953) had a male patient with the adult form, 2 of whose 4 sons had the infantile form. Dodge (1967) examining the blood groups of patients with this condition found a significantly low level of group A. It has occasionally been reported in association with other anomalies of gut innervation such as achalasia of the cardia (Blades *et al.*, 1957).

(a) Clinical features

In the infantile form the clinical presentation is of projectile vomiting with visible peristalsis and a palpable mass. At operation the mass is found to consist of a greatly enlarged pylorus which is extremely hard, the enlargement being due to hypertrophy and possibly hyperplasia of the circular muscle. Symptoms rarely occur before the third week of life, and it is known that the condition is not present at birth. Wallgren (1946) gave barium meals to 1000 new-born male infants, 5 of whom later developed hypertrophic pyloric stenosis and 995 of whom did not. In none of the 5 who did was there any preformed stenosis of the pyloric canal and the radiological appearances did not differ from the other 995.

Physiological studies on these infants have shown that in spite of the hypertrophy the pylorus retains a lumen. Atkinson *et al.* (1957) demonstrated that there was no zone of increased intraluminal pressure and therefore no organic obstruction. The radiological findings (Runström, 1939) are gastric dilatation with increased peristalsis and the pylorus itself shows a ribbon-like lumen 1–2 mm wide with no peristalsis. The affected segment is about 2–3 cm long and the emptying time of the stomach is $1\frac{1}{2}$–2 hours. There is thus only a relative slowing of gastric emptying. There is some evidence that partial degrees of the condition may occur in which there is a narrow canal and slow gastric emptying, but it is not severe enough to produce symptoms.

It is known that if the baby can be kept alive during the period of severe vomiting there is a tendency for the condition to improve spontaneously. This clinical improvement could be due to the increase in strength of the gastric contractions, following some hypertrophy, which can then force the bolus through the narrow lumen. Follow-up studies on patients treated medically showed that the canal became slightly wider and longitudinal rugae appeared (Runström, 1939). The gastric emptying time was still slightly increased until the child was about 4 years old when it became normal. In 1921 Thomson had noted that children who survived became symptom-free, but the pylorus remained thick. Armitage and Rhind (1951) described a patient who had had a gastro-enterostomy as a baby, and had to be operated on for a perforated anastomotic ulcer. The pyloric tumour was still present and the wall of the pylorus was grossly hypertrophied. After a Ramstedt operation the tumour disappears in about 3 months. Lumsden and Truelove (1958) traced 17 adults who had had hypertrophic pyloric stenosis as infants. They had no symptoms but there was some narrowing of the distal part of the pyloric canal.

(b) Adult cases

A number of cases have been reported in which hypertrophic pyloric stenosis has presented in adult life, the first by Cruveilhier (1835). The predominance of the male sex is not so striking in the adult cases. Du Plessis (1966) found the sexes equal, Hiebert and Farris (1966) had 64% female cases and Bateson *et al.* (1969) found 10 out of 17 were male. The macroscopic appearances of the pyloric tumour are similar to those in infants. It stops abruptly at the duodenal junction (North and Johnson, 1950), and extends about 3·4 cm along the greater curve and 2·5 cm along the lesser curve (Crymble and Walmsley, 1933). In the adult there is quite frequently an associated gastric ulcer (Craver, 1957; Du Plessis, 1966; Bateson *et al.*, 1969). This could well be related to delayed gastric emptying. The hypertrophic pylorus is about 1·2–2·0 cm thick, compared to the normal of about 0·4–0·7 cm. The orifice is reduced from 1·2–1·5 cm to less than 0·3 cm (Knight, 1961).

(c) Pathology

The main pathological change in hypertrophic pyloric stenosis, whether of children or adults, is thickening of the smooth muscle. This hypertrophy involves the circular and the longitudinal muscle (Cameron, H. C., 1925; North and Johnson, 1950; Roberts, 1959). If the condition has persisted for some time there may be some hypertrophy of the muscle in the body of the stomach related to increased peristalsis. Observations on the myenteric plexus have been numerous and varying, but the neurones are certainly not absent on paraffin sections in patients from Europe and North America. Cases of pyloric stenosis with a similar muscular abnormality have been reported from South America with loss of ganglion cells in adults (Raia, 1943; Raia *et al.*, 1956). In these patients there was also some inflammatory infiltration of the plexus and it is very probable that they were Chagasic.

Herbst (1934) found degenerated neurones and round cell infiltration in the infantile form of the disease. Alarotu studied the neurones in this condition in great detail (Alarotu and Christensen, 1949; Alarotu, 1956). Using a number of different staining techniques he thought that there was an increase in the number of dead and chromatolytic cells with disorganisation of ganglia and glial proliferation. Belding and Kernohan (1953) found only an occasional normal neurone, the others having undergone chromatolysis or were represented by ghosts. They thought that these changes were similar to those produced by vagal stimulation and were due to exhaustion. A noteworthy feature commented on by several writers is the immaturity of many of the neurones. Friesen *et al.* (1956) found that in the normal infant of 2–4 weeks there were many mature ganglion cells with abundant cytoplasm, prominent cell and nuclear membranes, and containing well-developed nucleoli, In hypertrophic pyloric stenosis the number of such cells were markedly reduced and many ganglia contained none at all. Roberts (1959) found that the ganglia were smaller than normal and the intervals between them greater. He also noted fewer well-differentiated cells but commented that if this were a maturation defect there would be a greater incidence in premature infants, which is not so. Friesen and Pearse (1963) did some histochemical studies on these small neurones and showed that they were enzymatically active and not dead cells. Their studies showed that they were immature rather than effete.

The most interesting and relevant investigation on infantile pyloric stenosis was done by Rintoul and Kirkman (1961). They showed that although the non-argyrophil cells were normal, there was an absence of argyrophil cells. They found only two in hundreds of sections. These authors say that many neuronal changes seen by other workers on paraffin sections are artefact. It is certainly true that many neurones can be seen in normal material which appear to show chromatolysis or cell shrinkage with poor histological detail.

Two cases of adult hypertrophic pyloric stenosis were studied on autopsy material. One patient had had a pyloroplasty 4 months previously and in the other case the tumour was an incidental finding. In the latter the tumour was very much larger than in the former.

In both cases neurones were present on paraffin section. A large number of thick silver-stained sections were taken and no argyrophil cells could be found in the pylorus, although normal numbers were present in the duodenum. In the first case some ganglia were replaced by schwann cells and contained argyrophil debris looking very much like the ganglia of the oesophagus in achalasia of the cardia.

Conclusion

It would appear probable that infantile hypertrophic pyloric stenosis is due to a maturation failure. Neuroblasts which should develop into argyrophil cells fail to do so and the pyloric pump mechanism does not function. At birth there are no symptoms because the pyloric orifice is wide enough for the stomach to empty by gravity. As the muscle of the canal hypertrophies, probably because it is denervated, the lumen becomes too small and obstruction occurs. If the child survives the acute episode without surgery the increase in size of the stomach and the strength of its contractions eventually becomes great enough to force the contents through the narrow lumen.

Cases occurring in adult life may be infantile in origin, but have not caused symptoms until a complication such as a gastric ulcer supervened. However in view of the marked difference in sex incidence between infantile and adult cases and the histological findings in the case described here, it is possible that there may be a condition arising *de novo* in adult life, which is of a similar nature to achalasia of the cardia.

9 The small intestine

(a) Anatomy

The small intestine consists of the duodenum, a curved retroperitoneal portion about 30 cm long and the jejunum and ileum. The two latter structures together measure about 5 metres, of which about $\frac{2}{5}$ is jejunum and $\frac{3}{5}$ ileum. The mucous membrane is very thick particularly at the upper end and is arranged in circular folds. These are known as Kerckring's folds and are 3–10 mm wide in the jejunum, but smaller and less conspicuous in the ileum, towards the end of which they disappear. This accounts for the fact that the jejunum is palpably much thicker than the ileum. The folds are permanent and do not iron out when the gut is thrown into villi which project into the lumen from the intestinal glands. The villi are covered with columnar epithelium and contain a lacteal at the centre. The function of the folds and villi is to slow down the progression of luminal contents and increase the area available for absorption. Beneath the mucosa is the lamina propria, which, apart from connective tissue and lymphatics, contains thin smooth muscle fibres from the muscularis mucosae. These extend to the tips of the villi, and when they contract they indent the epithelial surface, increasing still further the absorptive area and exerting a pumping action on the villi. The muscularis mucosae which lies beneath the lamina propria consists of two thin layers, the outer longitudinal and the inner circular. The submucosa contains the submucous nervous plexus, Brunner's glands in the duodenum and a number of lymph follicles. The latter are much more plentiful in the ileum where they are aggregated into Peyer's patches. The smooth muscle coats are fairly thin, the outer longitudinal being compact, but the circular layer is usually broken up into bundles.

The myenteric plexus lies directly on the longitudinal muscle as there is no intermuscular septum. The neurones are plentiful but they are predominantly argyrophobe. There are fewer argyrophil cells in this region than elsewhere and they appear to increase in numbers towards the distal ileum (Fig. 9.1). The mesh of the plexus is larger than in the colon and the lack of argyrphil cells results in paucity of the thick straight axons characteristic of the intrinsic neurones. Some of the intrinsic fibres show visible beading and are presumably sympathetic.

The sympathetic supply to the small intestine is profuse and comes from branches of the coeliac and superior mesenteric ganglia. The efferent fibres to these ganglia arise in the lowest five thoracic and the upper two lumbar segments. The nerves travel through the mesentery beside the

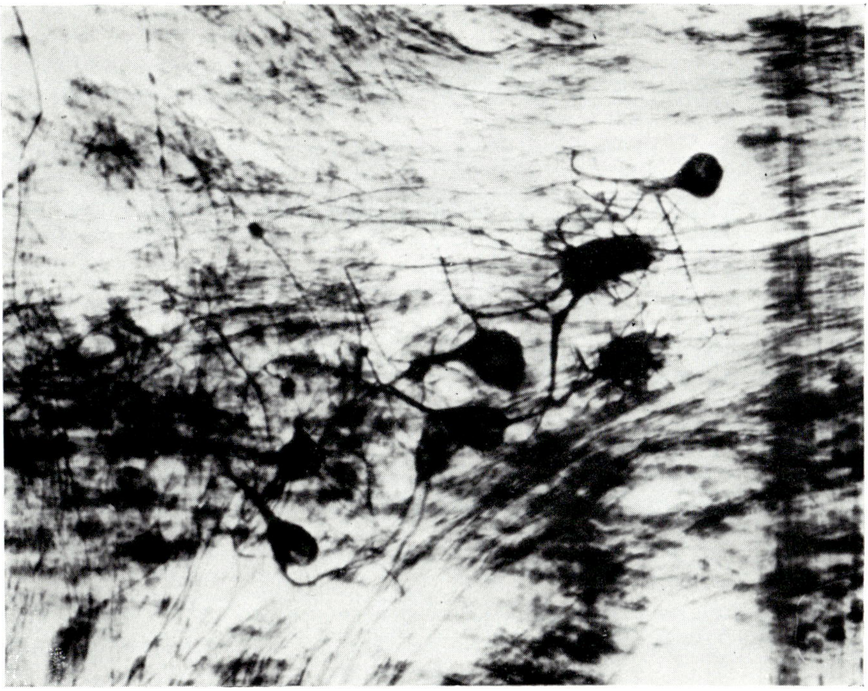

Fig. 9.1. The myenteric plexus of normal human ileum. The ganglion contains several multipolar cells of different shapes and one unipolar cell. Several of the neurones have more than one axon as well as a number of dendrites. The supporting schwann cells cannot be seen in a normal specimen.

blood vessels. The parasympathetic supply is usually considered to come from the vagus via the branch to the coeliac ganglion. This is a small nerve to supply such a large area of intestine in man. Patients rarely die following vagotomy, so it is not often possible to study the small intestine after this procedure. A boy of 7 with syringobulbia occupying the whole of the medulla died 6 weeks after developing dysphagia. Both vagi were destroyed as a result of damage to the dorsal vagal nuclei. A large number of fragmenting trunks were seen in the pylorus amounting to over $\frac{7}{8}$ of the total nerve supply. In the duodenum only 2 or 3 inches away the extrinsic innervation was virtually intact. Diligent search revealed three fragmenting axons out of many hundreds. This suggests that the vagal innervation beyond the pylorus may be rather scanty.

(b) Physiology

Movements of the small intestine have been observed by experimentalists for nearly a century. One early worker was Cash (1886) who noted that in the small intestine peristalsis was always aboral and proceeded at about 2 cm a minute. Mall (1896) described three types of contraction in the bowel wall. Firstly there were rhythmic contractions lasting about $5\frac{1}{2}$ seconds mainly in the circular muscle. Secondly there were vermicular contractions travelling down very fast through the whole intestine in about a minute. These seemed to be mainly seen in the dead animal. Thirdly there were propelling waves, always aboral and more rapid after a meal. They were more powerful in the duodenum than the ileum and were relatively inactive at night. If a segment of bowel were reversed surgically the wave moved oralwards. Bayliss and Starling (1899, 1900) used the dog, cat and rabbit. They described pendulum movements in which the longitudinal and circular muscle contracted together 10–12 times a minute. They travelled 2–5 cm a second and were myogenic in origin. Peristalsis was dependent on Auerbach's plexus and was always aboral. It was abolished by nicotine and cocaine. Local stimulation of the gut produced excitation above and inhibition below, a phenomenon which has become known as Starling's law of the intestine. They found that stimulation of the splanchnics inhibited both coats whereas vagal stimulation produced an initial inhibition followed by excitation.

Cannon (1901) used x-rays to follow the progress of bismuth in the dog's intestine. He saw rhythmical movements dividing the bolus into segments which were then redivided, the original cleavage lines rejoining. There was only a slight change in position of the bolus and the movements occurred 28–30 times a minute. There were two types of peristaltic wave, one advanced slowly for a short distance, the other moved rapidly through several coils. Cannon (1912) described the myenteric reflex. This is similar to Starling's law and shows contraction above and relaxation below the stimulated point. Segmentation was the local response to an increase in intraluminal pressure. In the cat he made incisions down to the submucosa at intervals of $1\frac{1}{2}$ to 2 cm for the first 45 cm of the bowel. This abolished peristalsis but had no effect on segmentation. Trendelenburg (1917) used the isolated guinea-pig ileum to show the peristaltic reflex. If the intraluminal pressure was raised a wave of contraction of the circular muscle layer passed aborally across the segment. Each wave of contraction was preceded by contraction of the longitudinal muscle, both layers relaxing simultaneously.

Carey (1921) suggested that nervous control was not necessary. Working with pigs he said that the circular and longitudinal muscles were both spirals. The inner coat was a tight spiral with a complete turn every $\frac{1}{2}$–1 mm, and the outer coat was an open spiral with a turn every 200–500 mm. He produced a mechanical model showing that such an arrangement could produce a differential rate of advance with cephalic constriction by the circular muscle and caudal dilatation by the longitudinal. This anatomy would account for the fact that the bolus progresses through the bowel in a spiral fashion moving in a counter-clockwise direction viewed from the cephalic end (Reid *et al.*, 1934). There is, however, good evidence that normal peristalsis is dependent on an intact innervation. Thomas and Kuntz (1926) showed that peristalsis was abolished by nicotine although segmentation persisted, and this has been confirmed by other workers. Peristalsis was unaffected by section of the vagus and sympathetic nerves 10 days previously (Bulbring *et al.* 1958). These same authors also showed that it could be abolished by asphyxia of the mucosa and the insertion of cocaine into the lumen. They suggested that the peristaltic reflex involved two sets of neurones, sensory to the mucosa and motor to the muscle coat. Certainly mechanical or inflammatory involvement of the mucosa, such as is produced by mercury purgatives or infection, results in a reflex increase in peristalsis probably via the submucosal plexus. Hukuhara, Sumi and Kotani (1961) destroyed the neurones in a loop of bowel by perfusing it with Tyrode solution for 4 hours. They said that this did not affect the muscle but destroyed the neurones with their higher oxygen consumption. The myogenic rhythmic contractions persisted.

An enormous amount of physiological and pharmacological work has been published on the intestinal smooth muscle, both in the intact animal and in isolated strips. The various active substances which are produced both in the normal and the pathological gut have been assayed and the effect of drugs on the muscle activity studied. This is very important from the point of view of our knowledge of smooth muscle function. It is also of clinical importance in that these active substances may alter the effectiveness of the neurotransmitter substance or the responsiveness of the muscle to the nervous impulse. This does not alter the fact that normal intestinal transit is dependent on a myenteric plexus which is intact anatomically. It may be possible to make the smooth muscle contract with drugs, but this does not ensure propulsion. If the plexus is badly damaged peristalsis cannot occur whatever pharmacological agents are applied.

10 The small intestine pathology

Chronic myenteric plexus damage in the small intestine is rare, but it does occur and it may be congenital or acquired. It affects a varying length of intestine which becomes dilated and grossly thickened. As has been discussed previously the plexus is not so important for transit in the small intestine as in the large and it is possible that short lesions produce no symptoms at all. In patients who do have symptoms these are frequently intermittent and even in the acquired cases go back many years. They are usually those of subacute intestinal obstruction with abdominal pain and vomiting. Laparotomies done every few years show only the dilated loop of bowel, without evidence of organic obstruction. This means little to a surgeon unfamiliar with the condition and either some sort of short circuit is done or no definitive procedure performed. Lack of medical understanding may result in the patient being labelled functional. A more serious aspect of the condition is that the aperistaltic segment, particularly if it is jejunal, acts as a 'blind loop', the contents stagnate and there is bacterial infestation and malabsorption. This malabsorption has been confused with the coeliac syndrome, but it does not respond to treatment by a gluten-free diet, and some patients have died from it.

The commonest region of the small intestine to be affected by a congenital abnormality of the plexus appears to be the duodenum. In these cases the duodenum is enormously dilated and thickened. It has been discussed clinically by several authors, although the disease is obviously rare (Corwin, 1915; Downes, 1917; Levin, 1923; Melchior, 1924; Jewett, 1928; Dudley, 1929; Nell, 1932; Kraas, 1933; Hunter, 1933; Petren, 1936; Weiss, 1938; Barnett *et al.*, 1955; Fisher, 1960). In the past the lesion was thought to be due to obstruction of the gut by the superior mesenteric vessels. Nell (1932), however, reported two cases in which the colon was not rotated, so that the mesenteric vessels did not cross the duodenum. Downes (1917) described a case of a boy of 4½, who had had intermittent vomiting since birth. At operation there was hypersegmentation of the gut wall and the duodenum was 3–4 times thicker than normal. Melchior (1924) first suggested that the term megaduodenum should be reserved for those cases with thickened walls without organic obstruction, to distinguish them from simple dilatation. He thought the condition was neurogenic. Hunter (1933) examined a still-born child with a distended abdomen. He found a grossly dilated duodenum and there were also dilations of three separate areas of ileum. Histology showed only traces of the myenteric plexus. Weiss (1938) described a case of a child with megaduodenum who also had Hirschsprung's disease. Two of his brothers had megaduodenum.

In some cases presenting in adult life the condition may or may not have been congenital. Barnett *et al.* (1955) described a female patient of 30 who had had attacks of vomiting for many years. She had hypertrophy of her duodenal wall and histology showed that it contained no neurones. Fischer (1960) surveyed a number of cases radiologically, one of which was known to have a thick muscle wall.

A condition which is sometimes associated with a very thick bowel wall is jejunal diverticulosis. One or two authors have thought that this could be due to neuromuscular imbalance. In 1881 William Osler described the post-mortem on a man of 65, who had 53 diverticula in the upper jejunum. This man's main complaint had been severe borborygmi. These had been so bad that he had to go out for a walk away from other people after a meal. Braithwaite (1923) reported a similar case of jejunal diverticula. There was an obvious increase in small intestinal motility and the jejunum was thick and dilated. This patient also would not sit in a room with other people after a meal. Edwards (1936) reviewed the pathogenesis of jejunal diverticulosis. He said that the diverticula were the result of mucosal herniation beside the blood vessels on either side of the mesenteric attachment. These gaps were closed when the muscle was contracted and widest when the muscle was relaxed. If the contraction was incoordinate it would be possible to have two contracted segments with a relaxed segment in between. The pressure in this relaxed area might be quite high and force the mucosa through the gap. This implies that some cases of jejunal diverticula have a neurogenic cause. Phillips (1952) described three further cases, all of whom had visible peristalsis and a thickened jejunal wall.

Acquired megaduodenum can occur in Chagas' disease. Raia *et al.* (1961) described 12 cases, all of whom had dilation of the duodenum with a thick muscle coat. There was incoordination of bowel movement and there were degenerative changes in the plexus. Three of these 12 cases had mega-oesophagus or megacolon in addition to the megaduodenum. The trypanosome can and frequently does affect the small intestine, but the signs and symptoms are usually overshadowed by colonic and oesophageal symptoms.

A condition has been described clinically in this country which may well be related to myenteric plexus damage. This is intestinal pseudo-obstruction. Naish *et al.* (1960) described a patient complaining of noisy abdominal colic, fatty diarrhoea, malabsorption and loss of weight, abdominal distension with audible and visible peristalsis, episodes of obstruction and marked segmentation movements of the gut visible clinically and radiologically. At his first laparotomy his appendix was removed, at his second 5 years later, a small abscess was found. At a barium meal the same year there was considerable dilution of the barium in the small bowel. Two months later the plain x-ray of the abdomen showed distended coils of small intestine. At his third laparotomy a month after this, gut movements were very active with hypersegmentation. A gluten-free diet did not improve his condition and he has continued to get intermittent pseudo-obstruction. The histology of the jejunum which was biopsied at the last operation, showed gross thickening of the inner muscle coat which was about 10 times thicker than the outer, the normal being 3 to 4 times. Dudley *et al.* (1958) reviewed a number of cases of intestinal obstruction in which no cause was found. In one patient the plain x-ray showed multiple fluid levels in the intestine.

A feature common to most cases is malabsorption, and this may be the presenting feature masking the motility problems. Ingelfinger (1943) reviewing non-tropical sprue had one patient with repeated subacute obstruction. He had two ileostomies, but his cramps and hypermotility persisted. Out of 100 patients with idiopathic steatorrhoea discussed by Cooke *et al.* (1953), 2 underwent laparotomy for obstructive symptoms. McClelland *et al.* (1962) had a patient with idiopathic steatorrhoea who was found to have 6 feet of dilated and hypertrophied jejunum at laparotomy. Histology showed smooth muscle hypertrophy, the fibres were 10–30 μ instead of 6 μ. Chesterman (1946) described 2 cases of obstruction for which no cause could be found. Naish *et al.* (1960) in addition to the case described above, mentioned 2 other cases with similar symptoms, one had the mucosal changes of the coeliac syndrome and the other a reticulosarcoma, probably only terminal.

The clinical and radiological picture of pseudo-obstruction seems to be readily recognisable. The pathological feature is the great thickening of the muscle coat; the plexus has not been examined.

Case report

The patient, a male storeman, developed intermittent epigastric pain, nausea and vomiting at the age of 48. Four years later a barium meal showed a small ulcer on the lesser curve of the stomach and some dilatation of the duodenum and upper jejunum. After a further four years he had a recurrence of symptoms with abdominal distension after meals, visible peristalsis and some weight loss. A laparotomy was done which showed no organic obstruction and no definite procedure was performed. The attacks of pain continued and the stools became bulky and offensive. At the age of 60 he had a further recurrence of pain and a second laparotomy was done. It was noted that the stomach, duodenum and upper jejunum were dilated and a posterior gastro-jejunostomy was performed. At the age of 65 he had a third laparotomy and this showed some hypertrophy of the duodenum and jejunum. A vagotomy was done. On admission a year later he had been bedfast for 7 months, he was wasted and dehydrated with a blood pressure of 95/65. There was abdominal distension, visible peristalsis and hyperactive bowel sounds. A barium meal showed stasis in the dilated upper gastrointestinal tract, some barium remaining

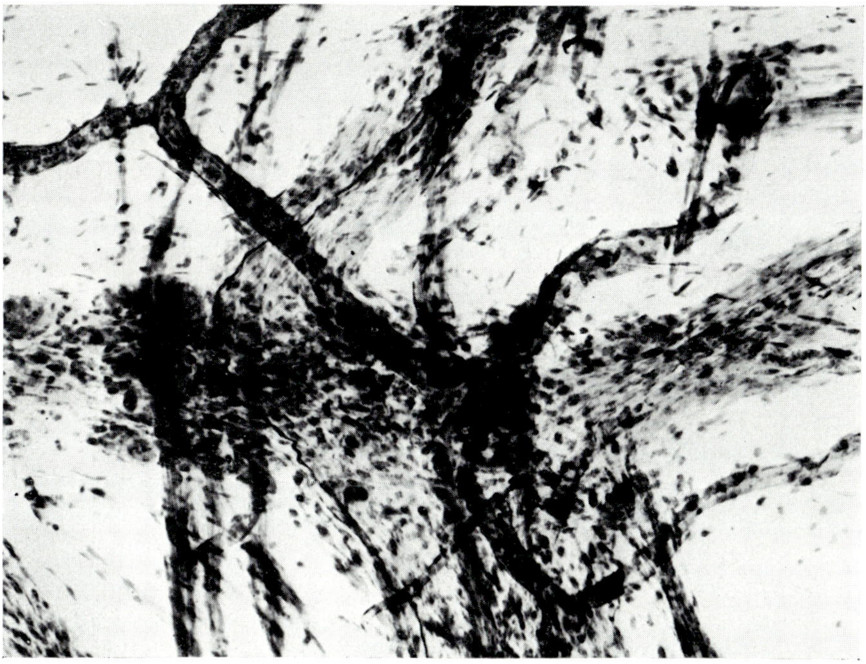

Fig. 10.1. The myenteric plexus of the ileum in a case of intestinal pseudo-obstruction. Only one neurone remains, which is larger than normal, and all its processes are truncated with swollen ends. The schwann cell proliferation can be seen in the background.

in the stomach and proximal jejunum for 24 hours. At a fourth laparotomy the stomach was enlarged and atonic. There was dilation of the jejunum and the wall was very thick. There was segmentation of the involved loop but no peristalsis. A sharp transition to macroscopically normal bowel was present in the lower jejunum. The third and fourth parts of the duodenum and 100 cm of jejunum were resected. An antrectomy was done and the stomach remnant anastomosed to normal jejunum. The second part of the duodenum was joined end-to-side to the jejunum at a lower level. In the succeeding 5 months the patient gained two stone in weight and remains symptom-free. However physical examination still shows a very noisy abdomen and it is likely that some aperistaltic gut remains.

Bacteriological investigation of the excised loop demonstrated a marked increase in micro-organisms. The paraffin sections confirmed the thickening of the smooth muscle, both inner and outer coats. The myenteric plexus contained a few macrophages and there was a little more collagen

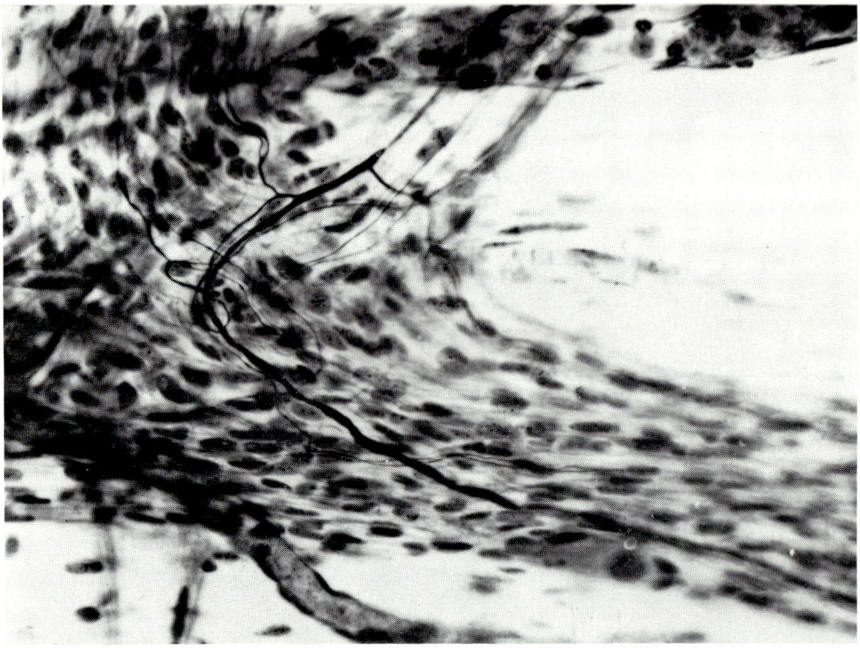

Fig. 10.2. The myenteric plexus of the ileum in a case of intestinal pseudo-obstruction. Part of the plexus is seen, largely replaced by schwann cells, but there is one residual axon and a number of branches.

present than normal. However ganglion cells were present, and it was not possible to detect fall-out with certainty. Silver preparations showed a very definite reduction in argyrophil neurones. Some of those which remained were very abnormal in morphology with swollen bodies and clubbed processes. Many axons were missing and there was a marked increase in the size and number of schwann cells (Figs. 10.1, 10.2 and 10.3). The damage was most severe at the distal end of the specimen, but there was some pathology in the duodenum.

Discussion

A feature of this case and of several described in the literature is the very long remittent history with negative or inconclusive laparotomies. In some cases the thick dilated bowel was noted and not removed. It is probable that, most of the time, the peristaltic activity of normal bowel above is sufficient to propel the liquid contents through the aperistaltic loop, although rather slowly. Every now and then there is a temporary hold-up

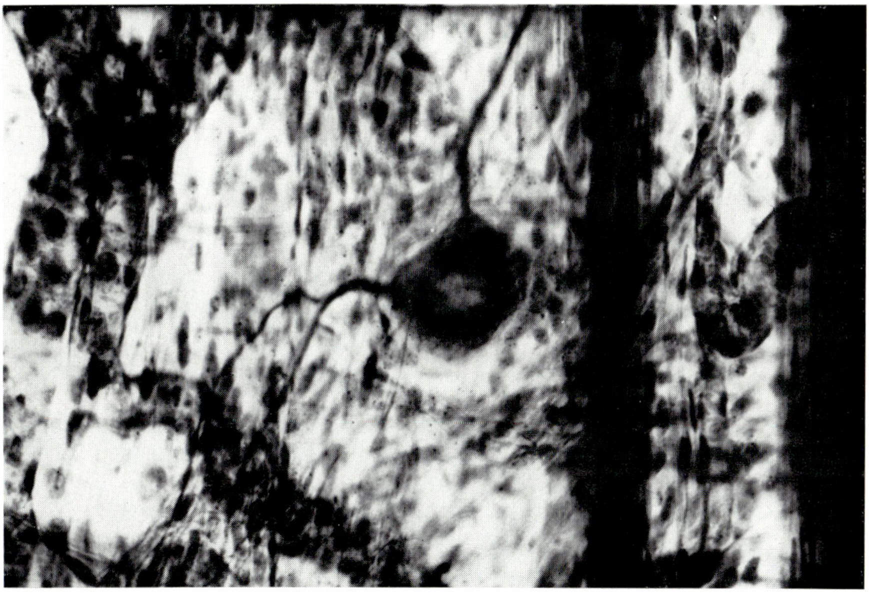

Fig. 10.3. The myenteric plexus of the ileum in a case of intestinal pseudo-obstruction. The ganglion is full of schwann cells and the remaining neurone is swollen and has lost its dendrites. Two axons are present, one of them branching.

with the production of colic and perhaps vomiting. The pain probably arises in the normal gut proximal to the lesion. The pain receptors to the intestine have not been identified, but in the oesophagus and the colon, lesions of the myenteric plexus are relatively painless, and it may be that they are involved in the disease process. In most cases it is the bacterial infestation of the aperistaltic loop with resultant malabsorption which seems to be the main cause of ill-health. The critical factor is probably the length of small intestine involved and this brings up the question of whether this is a progressive disease. The clinical histories suggest that this may be so, the absorption becoming worse and the attacks of colic more frequent as the amount of bowel involved increases. However the descriptions of the appearance of the intestine at laparotomy are not given in enough detail to know whether there is definite progression.

The only treatment of value is the administration of antibiotics and the removal of the denervated bowel as far as this is practicable. Even if, as in the case described here, some denervated bowel was not yet macroscopically thickened and therefore left behind, this may not matter clinically. Short stretches of bowel can be passed by the action of the normal gut above and the bacterial infestation will not be severe. Only if the disease progresses further will there be any need for further surgery. Subtotal removal may be enough if circumstances do not permit a complete excision.

This condition is not common, but once the aetiology is understood and the right treatment instituted the results may be dramatic.

11 The large intestine

(a) Anatomy

The colon is about 150 cm long and consists of ascending, transverse, descending and sigmoid portions. It is widest at the caecum and narrowest at the pelvi-rectal junction. The outer muscle coat is not uniform, but is divided into three bands or taeniae about 8 mm wide, the rest of the coat being very thin. These taeniae merge to form a continuous coat at the appendix and at the rectum. The taeniae are shorter than the rest of the bowel and pull it in into sacculations or haustrae. The more the taeniae contract, the more marked is the haustration. There are usually one or more rows of appendices epiploicae along the margins of the taeniae. The inner coat is continuous and similar to that in the small intestine. On the mucosal aspect the plicae semilunares correspond to the folds between the haustrae and unlike the folds of Kerckring include the muscle layer. The muscularis mucosae is relatively thin in this region and closely related to the mucosa. The mucous membrane does not contain villi, but has deep tubular pits going down to the muscularis mucosae. The epithelial cells are tall and prismatic and there are numerous goblet cells.

The extrinsic parasympathetic supply to the colon is partly derived from the vagus and partly from the sacral parasympathetic nerves, S2, 3 and 4. The former mainly supplies the midgut derivative and the latter the hind-gut. The junction point is somewhere near the splenic flexure, but there is considerable overlap. The vagal supply comes by the branch to the coeliac ganglion and travels along the mesentery, sometimes with the sympathetic trunks and sometimes separately, to the mesenteric border of the gut. The course of the sacral nerves has been a matter of some controversy. In 1934 Telford and Stopford described two bundles of nerve fibres on the ventral aspect of the hypogastric plexus, which converged and fused on the left side of the plexus. It then passed up over the left common iliac artery to the inferior mesenteric plexus. From thence the branches ran with the arteries to the bowel wall. Mitchell (1935) found the situation as described by Telford and Stopford in only 4 out of 15 cases. In most specimens there were several branches not just one from the hypogastric plexus. Three to ten nerves on each side left it for the colon. He suggested that the inferior mesenteric plexus was mainly or wholly sympathetic, and the hypogastric mainly parasympathetic. Woollard (1935) divided the pelvic nerves proximally in the cat and found no degenerated fibres in the hypogastric plexus. Lannon and Weller (1947) in a dissection of 9 Bantu infants, found the following situation. On the left side, fibres from the anterior sacral foraminae pierced the parietal layer of the pelvic fascia and immediately gave

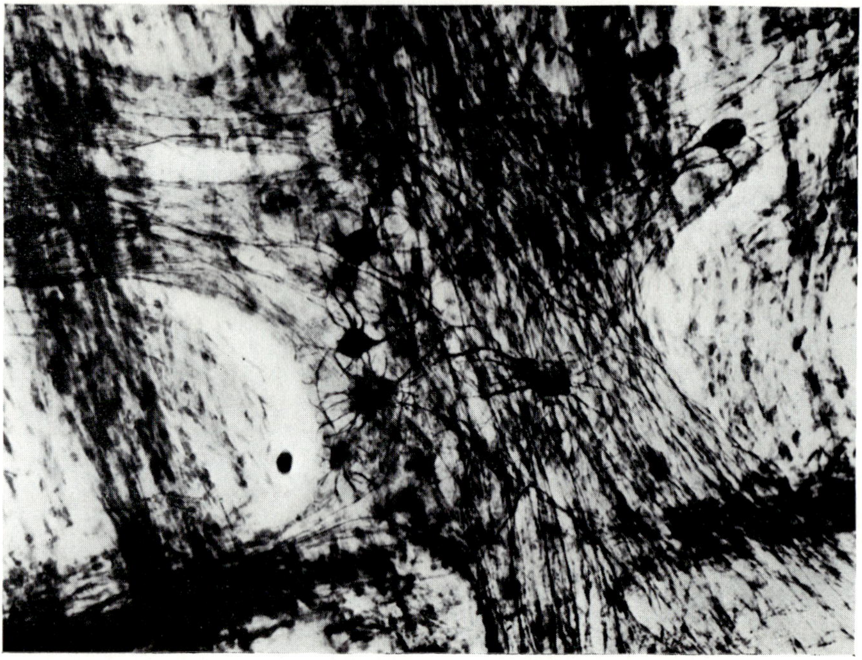

Fig. 11.1. The myenteric plexus of the normal human colon. The neurones are somewhat smaller and darker than elsewhere in the alimentary tract. Most of them are multipolar with thick relatively straight axons. The supporting schwann cells cannot be seen.

off a number of fibres to the rectum. The rest of the nerve became associated with the superior haemorrhoidal artery and communicated with the inferior hypogastric plexus. At the level of the sacral promontory the fibres swung away from the superior haemorrhoidal artery across the left common iliac artery into the mesentery. They did not accompany the blood vessels to the bowel, but crossed them obliquely. Fibres entering the colonic wall were traced as high as the middle of the descending colon.

On the right side the plan was similar, but the nerves lay further from the superior haemorrhoidal artery and closer to the hypogastric plexus. The fibres from the right side reached the intestine at a higher level than those of the left. Woodburne (1956) confirmed that the parasympathetic fibres ran diagonally to the inferior mesenteric system and entered the gut separately from the blood vessels. The parasympathetic nerves did not contribute to the hypogastric plexus, which is a wholly sympathetic structure.

The sympathetic supply to the colon is derived from the superior and inferior mesenteric ganglia. The segments of origin are from T10 in the caecum to L2 at the pelvi-rectal junction, and the peripheral distribution is similar to that in the small intestine. The rectum receives fibres from the hypogastric plexus.

There is no intermuscular septum in this region and the myenteric ganglia lie directly on the longitudinal muscle coat. They are more numerous beneath the taeniae than between them. The mesh of the plexus is relatively small and the fibre bundles are thick and straight. About 15–20% of the neurones appear to be argyrophil and they are very pleomorphic. Bipolar and unipolar forms are commoner in this region than elsewhere, and the shape may vary from oval to pyramidal to globular (Fig. 11.1). The extrinsic sympathetic supply appears less profuse here than it is in the small intestine and it is unusual to be able to pick out beaded sympathetic fibres within the plexus.

(b) Physiology

The colon is much less dynamic than the small intestine. Its movements were studied experimentally by Langley and Anderson in 1895. They noted that stimulation of the lumbar nerves produced pallor and inhibition of the muscle in the descending colon of cats, and if the sacral nerves were stimulated in the rabbit there was contraction of both muscle coats. In 1900 Bayliss and Starling, using mainly dogs, studied movements in anaesthetised animals. They isolated the colon by dividing the terminal ileum and rectum and placed it in a bath of warm saline. A balloon was placed in the lumen and attached to a recording tambour. They noted rhythmic contractions, each lasting only 2–4 seconds. Pinching the bowel produced inhibition of the entire colon below the point of stimulus. Stimulation of sympathetic nerves produced loss of tone and cessation of rhythmic contractions and this response was very difficult to fatigue. If the pelvic nerves were stimulated there was a slight initial relaxation, and then the whole gut contracted. This contraction was rather more marked distally than proximally. Cannon (1901) used bismuth subnitrate in animals and watched its progress by means of x-rays. He stated that the usual movement of the ascending and transverse colon was antiperistalsis.

It occurred about every 15 minutes and lasted about 5 minutes, the ileo-caecal valve preventing reflux. The movements continued during sleep but were inhibited by emotion. Elliot and Barclay-Smith (1904) used a similar technique to Bayliss and Starling, but first destroyed the spinal cord. They forced gruel into the ileum as a stimulus and noted waves of constriction running backwards to the caecum preventing further progress down the colon. There was a churning movement in the proximal colon which they said was a myogenic response to distension. Some coordinated peristalsis was seen in the transverse colon, which was inhibited by sympathetic stimulation. Stimulation of the pelvic nerves produced a strong contraction which emptied the distal colon. Much later Learmonth and Markowitz (1930) divided the lumbar colonic nerves and noted an increase in intra-colonic pressure and in the amplitude of the contractions. They considered that the sympathetic system exerted a constant inhibitory effect on the colon. In 1926 Welch and Plant introduced balloons into the colon of a number of dogs. The tracings showed that most of the time the gut was relatively inactive. About every 15–30 minutes there was a vigorous contraction and the number and size of these contractions were greater if the gut was distended. The ingestion of food increased this motility and even the entrance of the man who usually fed the dog. Templeton and Lawson (1932) distended the proximal colon of the dog with mineral oil, which produced a temporary increase in motility. In 1940 Adler and Templeton recorded from balloons placed in the dog's colon. The colon showed weak rhythmic contractions over the entire area or just the distal half. Sudden changes in the pressure waves were seen to move either analwards or oralwards. They considered that the weaker contractions corresponded to non-propulsive haustral segmentation and vigorous activity to mass movements.

Holznecht (1909) was the first man to study the human colon with x-rays. He noted mass movements in which the haustrae suddenly disappeared along the whole of the transverse colon, the ascending colon remaining unchanged. The transverse colon appeared quite smooth until the ribbon broke at the hepatic flexure and the contents were forced forward into the descending colon which had previously been empty. This process took about 3 seconds and after it was over haustral segmentation reappeared. Hertz (Hurst) and Newton (1913) undertook a similar investigation in normal subjects. They noted that the caecum filled in spurts from the ileum and the level in the caecum and the ascending colon rose passively. This filling was fastest after a meal because at that time the ileum was most active. The main movements of the large intestine were segmentation and compression of haustrae not associated with propulsion. These movements were small, rapid and present most of the time. Three or four times a day, usually after meals, there was a rapid mass movement in which faeces were propelled a considerable distance, the patient being unaware of this passage. Barclay (1935) used x-ray cinematography in patients who had been given bismuth pills coated with celluloid. These pills did not move onwards but in a more or less circular movement round the bowel. A patient with a paper-thin abdominal wall following excision of an epithelioma was described by Ghormley *et al.* (1954). They could see that non-propulsive haustration was the main movement. Propulsion only occurred after a meal and did not reach consciousness.

12 Chagas' disease

Chagas' disease is caused by the *Trypanosoma cruzi*, and is thus almost confined to South America, mainly Brazil, with a few sporadic cases being found in North America. It was first described by Chagas in 1910. It is rarely seen in Europe but it is of considerable importance, because according to the World Health Organisation (1960) there are 7 million cases in Latin America. It is also of interest because it is the only condition in which there is specific damage to the myxenteric plexus and the cause is known.

Chagas' disease is said to have been the cause of Charles Darwin's life-long indisposition. As a young man Darwin had been healthy and athletic, until about a year after he returned from the five-year voyage on the *Beagle*. He gradually gave up his energetic pursuits, including his field work, and when only thirty-three, he retired to his country house. He seldom went out, and relied on correspondence to keep up with scientific events. He had one illness on the *Beagle* when he was in Chile, which was said to have been typhoid. Saul Adler (1959) has said that in March 1835, in the Argentinian province of Mendoza, Darwin was bitten by the benchuca, *Triatoma Infestans*. If this were so, the chances of infection by the trypanosome were very high. A point against the infective theory is that there appears to have been no acute fever or lymphadenopathy. However, this, apparently, is not all that uncommon and in quite a number of cases the onset is just another insect bite with no symptoms, until heart failure or some other complication supervenes. He also survived another forty years in spite of his symptoms. This is a longer life span than is usual in this disease.

The trypanosome is spread by an insect vector, the Reduviid bug, either *Triatoma Infestans* or *Panstrongylus Geniculatus*. The bug is infected by biting animals; armadilloes, monkeys and opossums are common reservoirs, but others, including the domestic cat and dog, can act as such. It lives in the cracks in the walls of houses whence it emerges to feed. The trypanosome is produced in the intestine of the triatome and excreted in the faeces. Human infection occurs from rubbing the faeces into a bite, usually on the face. The insect is sometimes known as the 'kissing' bug from its tendency to bite around the mouth. This produces severe local oedema and is followed by a generalised infective process with fever, lymphadenopathy, hepato-splenomegaly and occasionally a fatal meningitis. The trypanosomes enter the blood stream and invade tissue cells, where they become leishmanias with large nuclei and blepharoplasts. The leishmanias divide inside the cells to form small colonies and frequently produce necrosis. Particularly in muscle this necrosis may be associated with an acute inflammatory response. In other cases the leishmania colony may form a small cyst around itself. Usually the infestation tends to die out in the course of time, and the patient is left with the results of the damage in the heart and alimentary canal.

The diagnosis can be made by examining the serum, skin or lymph node biopsies for the organism. In the early stages, before the infection is widespread, it may be made by allowing uninfected bugs to feed on the patient, and then examining their stools two or three weeks later (Brumpt, 1914). A complement-fixation test was introduced by Machado Guerreiro using either a culture of *T. cruzi* or infected animal tissue as antigen.

The relation between the trypanosome and the disease has been further demonstrated by Okumura and Neto (1961), who injected the organism into a number of laboratory animals. They showed that the organism lived in the walls of viscera and suggested that it produced a toxin which destroyed ganglion cells. There is no treatment, as yet, for the infection, and the only procedure of value is to try and keep down the vector.

The most important aspect of the disease is the chronic stage. Although theoretically any organ may be affected, in practice the heart, the oesophagus and the colon are most frequently involved clinically. Of these the heart has been the most thoroughly investigated (Laranja *et al.*, 1956; Köberle, 1963). The patients have right bundle branch block, and the heart progressively enlarges, often reaching a weight of 600 to 700 grams, until they ultimately die of heart failure.

The gastrointestinal involvement is manifested clinically by dysphagia and constipation, and pathologically by enteromegaly. The incidence is high. In São Paulo, megacolon was found in 69 out of 556 consecutive autopsies (Ferreira-Santos and Carril, 1964). Most patients seem to put up with the chronic ill-health associated with the disease unless they come to surgery either for severe dysphagia or volvulus of the enormous sigmoid colon. Köberle (1957, 1963) has shown that the lesion in the oesophagus and in the colon is associated with a loss of myenteric neurones. Vieira *et al.* (1964) demonstrated that gut removed surgically from patients with Chagas' disease was hypersensitive to cholinergic drugs. This they ascribe to the hypersensitivity of denervated structures.

Three colonic cases studied pathologically varied somewhat in the extent of the disease. The bowels were all dilated, up to 18 cm maximum circumference, and showed little evidence of haustration. The muscle although an occasional nucleus of an argyrophobe cell could be seen. In most sections the loss of argyrophil cells was complete, but that of argyrophobe cells less so. Where argyrophil cells could be identified they were very abnormal, with swollen and irregular processes (Fig. 12.2). Another feature was the presence of single aberrant fibres in the muscle coats away from the plexus. These were very thick and of uniform calibre, and had the appearance of parasympathetic fibres. They could have been extrinsic fibres which had been damaged distally by the inflammatory process and lost their effector neurones, growing aimlessly through the muscle. It is also possible that they were the axons of surviving intrinsic neurones, but this is unlikely as none were seen with normal processes.

These cases illustrate well the effect of myenteric plexus destruction on the intestinal wall. The colon is dilated and grossly thickened. There is an increase in intestinal mass, and it is thus a true 'megacolon' in contradistinction to cases to which this label is frequently applied, which are simple dilations. There is hypertrophy of the smooth muscle with active nuclei, and it is possible that there is also hyperplasia. The cause of this has been discussed in Chapter 3, p. 16.

13 Acquired megacolon

Acquired damage to the colonic myenteric plexus, which is not due to drugs or to Chagas' disease, has rarely been demonstrated histologically. Clinically constipation is such a common complaint, nearly all of it functional, that it is extremely difficult to extract from this morass the very occasional patient who would benefit from surgical treatment. From the days of Arbuthnot Lane who removed a very large number of intestines with a 28% mortality, the pendulum has swung right back. Surgeons are now very unwilling to do any operative procedure just because the patient has to have enemas to empty his colon. Until there is good physiological and histological evidence that the plexus is irretrievably damaged this is likely to remain so, although nowadays the mortality from partial colectomy is very low in the hands of the rectal surgeons.

Histological investigation of 20 cases of colectomy, done for constipation of unknown origin, showed the following findings. Twelve had no significant abnormality, 5 showed damage due to excessive use of purgatives but 3 showed a lesion which could be distinguished from that due to cathartics and was somewhat similar to that seen in myenteric plexus disease in the small intestine.

The first patient was a woman who had developed constipation in her early teens. By the time she was 26, it had become worse and responded poorly to aperiants. At the age of 28 she was beginning to get attacks of colic, nausea and vomiting and a barium enema showed no abnormality. She was, however, unable to evacuate the barium. Physiological studies three years later suggested failure of propulsion and a balloon in the rectum could be filled with 700 ml of fluid before the anal sphincter relaxed. She was unable to defaecate the balloon. A transverse colostomy was made which functioned well. A Duhamel procedure was done and the colostomy closed, but following this she became constipated again. She was admitted twice in the following 6 months with faecal impaction. A sigmoid colostomy was done which failed to function without excessive purgative administration. Finally a further excision was done and the colon removed back to the region of the original transverse colostomy, which had been known to work, and a transverse-rectal anastomosis done. Now, 2 years later, she is well and having her bowels open normally. There is, however, some abdominal distension clinically, and it is possible either that the disease process is progressive or that some denervated gut remains behind.

The second patient was a woman of 47 who had suffered increasing constipation for many years. Eight years previously she had had a rectal prolapse repaired and three years previously her transverse and descending colon were removed. This specimen was not available for study. The operation did not improve her symptoms and all faeces had to be removed manually. A further excision was done and an ileo-rectal anastomosis performed. This relieved her constipation but she still has some colicky abdominal pain, so she may have some pathology in the small intestine.

The third patient was a woman of 54. It is not clear from the history how long she had been constipated, but for five years she had had to have bowel wash-outs and had not had a normal action. A left-sided colectomy was done but it is too early to say how useful this has been.

Examination of the surgical specimens showed, in both samples from the first case, some dilatation, the maximum circumference being 14–15 cm, and some generalised thickening of the muscle coats, particularly the inner. In the second case the thickening was somewhat patchy and there were one or two thin areas. In the third case only three small random samples were available, one of which was thicker than normal. Thin paraffin sections showed some increase in macrophages in a few ganglia in case 1 but little else significant. It was not possible to say that the ganglion cells were reduced.

The silver preparations, which were of course much thicker, showed one or two ganglia in case 1 to be replaced by inflammatory cells. Otherwise the changes were similar in the three cases. There was a definite loss of argyrophil cells and many of the ones which remained showed a characteristic change. They were swollen and slightly paler than normal, the silver-positive material giving a speckled appearance instead of being uniformly black. The edges of the cell were indistinct and the processes paler and much thicker than normal. There was an increase in number and size of schwann cells in the ganglia but it was less apparent in the nerve trunks. Many ganglia appeared to contain no neurones at all and it is probable that there was a reduction in argyrophobe cells as well. In case 1 a few ganglia were necrotic containing only axonal debris.

These cases show evidence of organic plexus damage with thickening of the smooth muscle. Two of them have done well following surgery and the fate of the third is not yet established. It is impossible to tell from the clinical literature how common the condition is. Cases of megacolon are described, but in many instances this merely implies dilatation of the gut. This, of course, can be enormous, particularly in the sigmoid with or without symptoms. Histology of such cases, including that from a woman of 80 whose sigmoid colon had a circumference of 48 cm, show only changes due to stretch. This particular patient had had a couple of attacks of volvulus and she appears to have died from fluid loss into this enormous structure, but she had had no motility problem. Megacolon is also frequently reported in inmates of mental hospitals. Johnston and Gibson (1959) reported three cases. In the first the excised bowel did not respond to nicotine, but histologically ganglion cells were present. In the second case the myenteric plexus was normal at post-mortem and the third was similar to the first. The bowel was thickened in all cases. The failure to respond to nicotine in two instances strongly suggests that the neurones were unable to function. In a mental hospital population the most likely cause of this is therapy. The majority of drugs used to treat disturbed patients are anti-cholinergic, and if they have to be given for long periods of time they will eventually damage the myenteric neurones. Animal experiments suggest that this damage is unlikely to be detectable on standard histological preparations. However a single case was reported by Burrell (1957) in which there was thickening of the bowel wall and no neurones were seen.

The aetiology of the damage in the three cases described above is obscure and drugs were not a factor. Erskine (1963) reported a single case of a patient with dysphagia who had to have a cardiomyotomy. At the age of 30 she developed total constipation and at colectomy the gut was found to be very thick and dilated. Histologically there was lymphocytic infiltration and fibrosis of the plexus region and ganglion cells were scanty. The patient had not been out of the United States and the complement-fixation test for Chagas' disease was negative. However cases of Chagas' disease have been reported from North America and the findings were very suggestive of this condition as the author stated. The three cases described above would also be compatible with Chagas' disease. It has not been reported in England and no patient has been out of Europe. In one case the complement-fixation test for Chagas' disease was negative. It could, however, be due to an infective agent which behaves in a similar manner to the *T. cruzi*.

Most gastro enterologists have patients who appear to be unable to have a normal bowel action, although they are usually jollied along with purgatives and weekly enemas. This is a poor sort of life, and it might well be that in some cases surgery is justifiable. The major difficulty is to diagnose the organic nature of the condition before resection. At the moment physiologists are unable to say for certain whether there is peristalsis in the large bowel or not, although they can give other contributory information. It might help to solve the problem if all patients coming to colectomy for constipation had physiological studies performed first and histology done afterwards, so that the two can be correlated. A pattern of colonic behaviour might well emerge which would be of diagnostic significance.

14 Hirschsprung's disease

(a) Incidence

Hirschsprung first gave an account of the dilatation and hypertrophy of the colon in the new-born in 1888, and following this there were a number of European publications of single cases (Tittel, 1901; Brentano, 1904; Finney, 1908; Schmidt, 1909). Dalla Valle (1920) appears to have been the first writer to notice that the ganglion cells were absent, and also that the disease had a familial incidence. In 1928 Cameron described a case in which the ganglia were replaced by inflammatory cells similar to the picture described by Hurst and Rake (1930) in achalasia of the cardia. This is not the usual finding, and it is not at all certain if, in fact, it was Hirschsprung's disease. Definite studies of a series of cases were not made until 1948 by Whitehouse and Kernohan, and in 1949 by Bodian and his co-workers, although an accurate description of a single case was given in 1938 by Robertson and Kernohan. This latter appears to be the first description in English. Tiffin *et al.* (1940) reported a case with absent neurones in the sigmoid colon and noted an abundance of nerve fibres. The previous literature on the clinical aspects of the disease has been reviewed by Ehrenpreis (1946).

The condition is not very common and in the usual short segment cases, in which there is no disease proximal to the sigmoid colon, males appear to predominate very considerably. Whitehouse and Kernohan (1948) had 10 males and 1 female; Bodian *et al.* (1949), 36 boys and 3 girls. Nixon (1964) reported a male to female ratio of 5 : 1 and Gordon *et al.* (1966) 4·9 : 1. In the long segment cases in which the disease extends proximal to the sigmoid colon, the sex difference is not so marked. Nixon (1964) found that the incidence was the same in the two sexes and Gordon *et al.* (1966) found a male to female ratio of 1·6 : 1 in 18 cases.

Several authors have described a pronounced familial incidence of Hirschsprung's disease, particularly in the long segment cases. Bodian and Carter (1963) found that in the short segment cases the disease occurred in 1 in 20 of male siblings and 1 in 100 of female siblings, whereas in the long segment cases the incidence was 1 in 10 irrespective of sex. Fock and Kostia (1963) recorded the incidence of long segment disease in a brother and sister. They said that, at that time, there were 20 families in the literature in which 61 members had suspected or confirmed Hirschsprung's disease, $\frac{2}{3}$ of them males. Gordon *et al.* (1966) had one family in which there were two long segment cases in two sisters and another in a male cousin. Among their 56 studied cases there were 3 first cousin marriages. Passarge (1967) described 63 cases in which the 55 male examples had 2, possibly 3, affected siblings and 118 normal ones. The 8 female cases had 2 affected and 21 normal siblings. The 63 cases had 6 first cousins affected. Of 6 long segment cases, 2 had affected siblings who were also long segment.

In addition to its familial incidence, Bodian and Carter (1963) found a significant association of congenital megacolon with increasing maternal age, but Gordon *et al.* (1966) noted that in their patients, the mean maternal age was 28·7 years and paternal age 32·5 years. This is only about a year above the average for this racial group. It also has a relationship with Down's syndrome. De Wolff (1964) found 7 cases of Hirschsprung's disease, 4 confirmed at autopsy, among 134 children with Down's syndrome. Emanuel *et al.* (1965) reported 2 further cases of the association and suggested that mongols with severe constipation, which is very common, should be investigated for Hirschsprung's disease. Graivier and Sieber (1966) found Hirschsprung's disease in 3 out of 84 mongols and Passarge (1967) 6 out of 63. Gordon *et al.* (1966) found 1 case of Down's syndrome among 56 cases of congenital megacolon. The association between the two conditions does not appear to be a matter of chance, but although it has been suggested that an abnormality of chromosome 21 produces Hirschsprung's disease, no definitive chromosome studies appear to have been published yet.

Megacolon also occurs in some strains of laboratory mice. Derrick and Grambauer (1957) found 98 cases in about 20,000 mice. The distal colon had an undilated segment stretching 3 to 17 mm from the anus. There were firmly packed faeces above and some dilatation of the ascending colon and caecum. Histology showed absent ganglion cells and bundles of unmyelinated fibres. In another strain of mice a similar condition was found to be associated with recessive spotting genes (Lane, 1966). The author suggested that this might be due to the fact that skin pigmentation and the intestinal nerve supply were both related to the neural crest. Bielschowsky and Schofield (1962) also showed aganglionosis in a strain of piebald mice with megacolon. These writers considered that it was a degenerative condition with loss of neurones rather than congenital absence.

(b) Clinical features

The clinical features of Hirschsprung's disease in man vary with the severity of the condition and particularly with the length of the aganglionic segment. It is a congenital condition, and symptoms always start from birth. In the severe cases the presentation is of neonatal intestinal obstruction, only relieved by colostomy or even ileostomy. The mortality is about 50% in the first year of life. The passage of the first meconium stool is delayed for several days and is followed by constipation, gaseous abdominal distension and usually vomiting. This may come in attacks, but in between these attacks the child shows chronic abdominal enlargement. Flatus is passed frequently, and a striking feature is the absence of any abdominal pain in the attacks. The faeces are usually small and rabbity or tooth-past-like ribbons. Later the chronic distension is associated with visible peristalsis. On examination the rectum is empty. In milder cases there are no acute episodes, but the child presents with a distended abdomen and wasted buttocks. These children are prone to infection both of the gut and of the respiratory system. Some patients do manage to get through childhood and do not come to surgery until adult life. When going into their history, it is apparent that they have had symptoms since birth, and have never enjoyed good health. In a 10-year period, 16 cases of adult Hirschsprung's disease were operated on at St. Mark's Hospital. This represents about a quarter of the total number of cases of megacolon seen during that period (Jennings, 1967). An additional complication which may occur in untreated cases is an entercolitis from which no pathogenic bacteria have been isolated. It results in severe diarrhoea which may be fatal in young children if not treated swiftly.

(c) Radiology

The radiological findings in this condition are diagnostic, but not always easy to demonstrate. Once there is a lot of barium in the dilated portion, the picture is obscured. The bowel should not be prepared, but a small amount of barium run in under visual control. As soon as it is observed entering the dilated portion no more is given. Large amounts of barium increase the patient's symptoms, and water may be absorbed so quickly from the dilated bowel that water intoxication follows. The rectum is seen to be of normal or less than normal size. Above this the gut narrows for a variable distance, usually less than 12 inches, and then opens into a very wide funnel. There is no visible muscular contraction in the narrowed segment.

(d) Treatment

The treatment of Hirschsprung's disease is excision, with or without a preliminary colostomy. Svenson and Bill (1948) concluded that the narrow spastic segment was causing the obstruction and removed this segment by a pull-through technique, with preservation of the sphincter. This is still the standard procedure in some centres. Its disadvantages are that it has a rather high complication rate of stricture and incontinence. If the rectum is removed, the bowel which replaces it does not have normal rectal sensation and control may be difficult. There is also the danger of interfering with the nerve supply of the bladder. A number of modifications have been introduced, the most important being that by Duhamel (1959). The upper end of the rectum is divided and closed, the aganglionic segment is excised, and the proximal colon drawn down behind the rectum and out through the posterior half of the anus between the external and internal sphincters. Crushing clamps are then applied, converting the rectum and colon into a single chamber with normal rectal sensation anteriorly and propulsive colon posteriorly.

(e) Pathology

Whitehouse and Kernohan (1948) studied 11 cases, 10 post-mortem and 1 which had been resected surgically. They used 78 normal intestines as controls and established that ganglion cells were present in every section taken from normal colon. So-called degenerative changes in the neurones were commonly seen in both patients and controls. Non-myelinated nerve trunks in the location of the plexus were rare in the colon and rectum. Extreme dilatation of the colon had little effect on the appearance of the plexus. The rectum contained as many ganglia as other parts of the large intestine or more. They did not note the separation of ganglion cells into Dogiel type 1 and 2 and made no comment about the nature of the interstitial cells. These authors used the Bodian silver method on paraffin sections cut transverse to the gut.

In the patients with Hirschsprung's disease no ganglion cells were present in the distal colon and the population in the descending colon was normal. In between, somewhere in the sigmoid and varying from case to case, was a transitional zone. In every case there were non-myelinated nerve trunks between the circular and longitudinal muscle layers, which were not present in the controls. The authors were not impressed by any degenerative change in the neurones which were present and could find no evidence of inflammatory change.

Bodian *et al.* (1949) studied 15 specimens, 2 from post-mortems and 13 from surgical resections. They found complete absence of ganglion cells throughout the narrowed segments and extending 1–5 cm into the dilated segments. In the pathological areas there were numerous bundles of nerve fibres, but there were no inflammatory changes. The length of the affected segment varied, some included only the rectum and others a considerable part of the sigmoid. In one case it extended to the splenic flexure. Proximal to the pathological portion ganglion cells were normal in appearance but rather scanty.

A recent contribution to the pathology was made by Bennett *et al.* (1968) who demonstrated a great increase in the sympathetic innervation

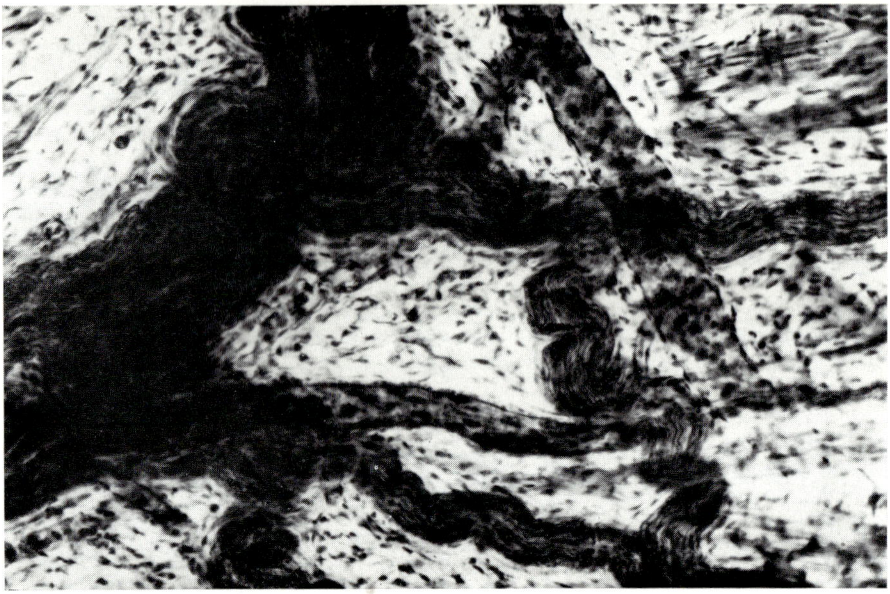

Fig. 14.1. The myenteric plexus from the contracted distal segment of a patient with Hirschsprung's disease. The normal plexus is replaced by an unmyelinated fibre network containing no neurones but similar in general lay-out to the normal plexus. These fibres are strongly cholinergic.

in the gut wall in the contracted segment of Hirschsprung's disease. Much of it appears to be in the muscle coats. As there are no neurones in this region, there can be no perineural synapses, and it is possible that in the absence of their normal terminations, the sympathetic fibres continue to grow.

(f) Present series

A study was made of the myenteric plexus in 7 cases of Hirschsprung's disease, 6 adults and a child. There were 5 males and 2 females. All the patients had a Duhamel type procedure and they have all done well following surgery. The adult specimens were 30–40 cm long. In the child the disease extended proximally into the transverse colon and he had to have a colostomy at 6 weeks of age, the final operation being done at 6 months.

Macroscopically all the specimens consisted of a contracted and a dilated portion, but the former was relatively short in the 6 adult cases.

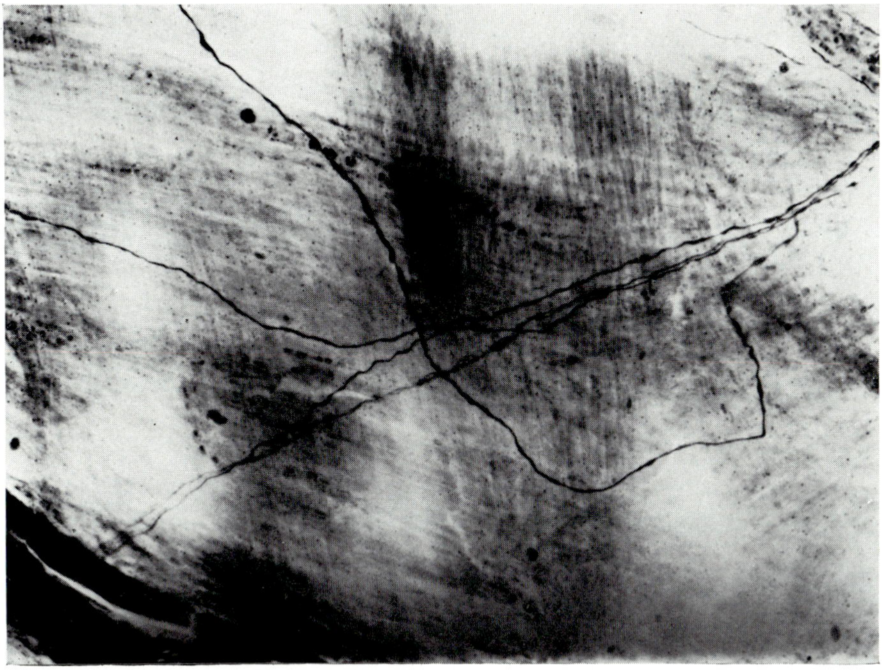

Fig. 14.2. Part of the circular muscle from the distal contracted segment of a patient with Hirschsprung's disease. It shows the single fibre network lying outside the area of the myenteric plexus. This is probably the adrenergic network which has been demonstrated in this region.

This is probably the most important reason why they did not have to undergo surgery in childhood. Both the contracted and dilated portions had considerable thickening of the smooth muscle coats. Paraffin sections in 5 cases showed no neurones in the contracted segment and replacement of the plexus by unmyelinated nerve fibres. In 2 cases a few neurones could be seen on all sections, although there were abnormalities, and unmyelinated nerve trunks were seen.

The silver preparations were similar in all 7 cases and quite characteristic of the disease. In the distal contracted segment, the nerve cells were scanty or absent. Those which were present were frequently abnormal in shape and had no processes. The striking feature was the presence of the branching system of unmyelinated nerve bundles. They consisted of fine wavy fibres packed closely together in contrast to the normal thick, straight, widely spaced axons. These bundles were arranged in a type of network which in places was somewhat similar to the pattern of the normal plexus

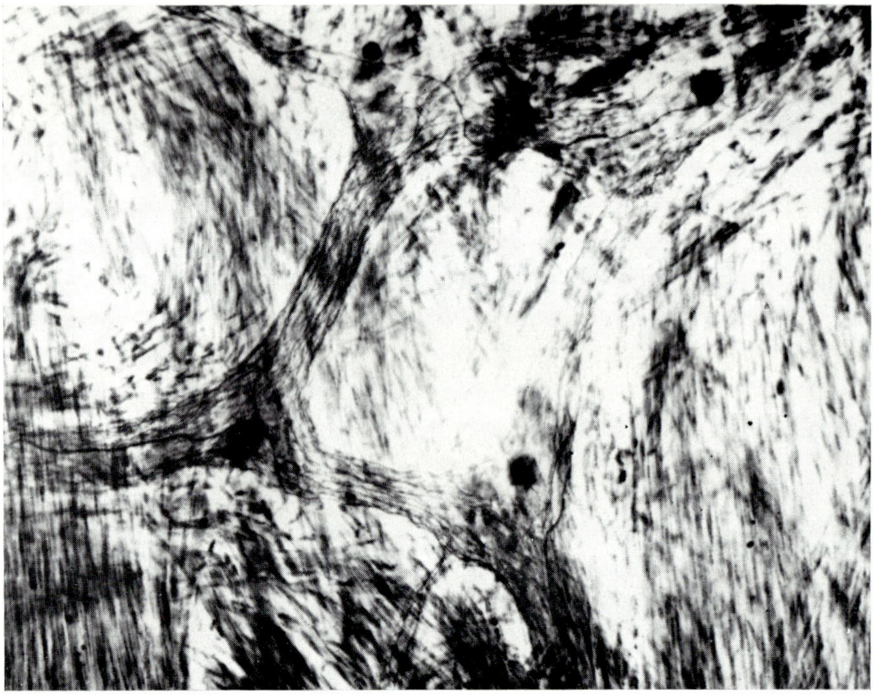

Fig. 14.3. The myenteric plexus from the proximal dilated portion of the colon of a patient with Hirschsprung's disease. The unmyelinated fibre network can still be seen, but neurones are beginning to appear at the angles. The ganglion cells themselves show poor morphology and few if any processes. These cells would, however, appear normal on a conventionally stained paraffin section.

(Fig. 14.1). In 3 cases, away from the plexus region in the circular muscle, there was a network of single fibres which were thick and slightly beaded (Fig. 14.2). These were almost certainly the abnormal sympathetic fibres demonstrated by Bennett *et al.* (1968) using the fluorescent catecholamine technique.

Sections taken from the dilated segment and the junction zone were rather variable. The number of neurones increased, but they continued to be very dark, rounded and with poorly formed processes. The unmyelinated nerve trunks could still be seen, but usually only short lengths and in some places the contained axons were themselves fragmented. The same trunks were seen to contain axons, often short, of intrinsic neurones. In 1 case a remaining portion of the unmyelinated nerve network was shown to be partially fragmented and to contain poorly formed neurones at the angles (Fig. 14.3). The lower fibres of the myenteric plexus proper were scanty, very thick and irregular in calibre. They did not show the normal geometrical pattern, but wandered in a random fashion, sometimes terminating abruptly and sometimes showing retraction balls (Plate II.1, facing p. 80). In no specimen was the plexus normal, even at the upper end. The gradation between the findings in the contracted portion and the dilated portion was not regular and sometimes proximal blocks were more abnormal than more distal ones. In particular small lengths of myelinated nerve trunks were scattered in a random fashion throughout the proximal part of the specimen.

In summary the features are replacement of the plexus in the contracted segment by unmyelinated fibre networks, and anatomical abnormalities of the plexus in the dilated segment right up to the upper cut end.

These findings show that the dilated segment, which has a very thick smooth muscle coat, has an incomplete and inadequate nerve supply. It is possible that some changes, particularly the retraction balls, are secondary to the dilatation of the gut, but this would not account for the anatomical abnormalities. The layout of the plexus is quite different from the normal and from that in which the lesion of the plexus is an acquired one, indicating that it was never formed correctly. Physiological studies by Zuelzer and Wilson (1948) in which they measured pressures through colostomy openings, suggest that there is hypersegmentation of the dilated portion This could be associated with impaired peristalsis for the same reason that it occurs in acquired enteromegaly as is discussed elsewhere (Chap. 3, p. 16).

Examination of surgical specimens pharmacologically has been done by Trounce and Nightingale (1960). They found that nicotine applied to the specimen would produce acetylcholine release and a contraction of the muscle. Wright and Shepherd (1965) found little difference from normal in the dilated portion of the bowel. In the contracted segment there was less response to acetylcholine, and it was contracted not relaxed by nicotine and DMPP (dimethylphenylpiperazinium). The bowel wall in Hirschsprung's disease is very thick compared to the normal, and may not respond quite so well in the pharmacological bath. If cholinergic nerves are present they may produce acetylcholine when stimulated and that acetylcholine may produce smooth muscle contraction, but if the anatomical connections of the neurones are awry there will be no coordinated movement. In the large bowel what matters clinically is not whether the smooth muscle is or is not capable of contraction under certain stimuli, but whether there is organised peristalsis. This is dependent not only on acetylcholine-producing neurones, but on their correct anatomical relationship and communication with the plexus and with each other. If this is abnormal the patient is unable to have his bowels open naturally.

(g) The relation of symptoms to pathology

The cause of the constipation in Hirschsprung's disease is usually considered to be obstruction by the contracted segment. It is true that the lumen is narrowed but it is far from completely obstructed and one would expect a normally active colon to force even solid contents through. In many cases the contracted segment is very short but the patients still have symptoms. It is apparent from the pathology that the dilated segment does not have a normal nerve supply or normal peristalsis. This is the reason why the partial obstruction cannot be overcome. The very thick wall and hypersegmentation of the dilated segment are additional features of the poor innervation. It is worth noting that some abnormal bowel remained behind in all these patients who, nevertheless, did very well after surgery. With relief of the partial obstruction the peristaltic action of normal bowel proximally is adequate to pass the aperistaltic segment which could be quite short. Experience with other cases suggests that short aperistaltic segments are passed easily and that there is probably a critical length, both in the large and small intestine, above which symptoms may occur.

(h) The development of the myenteric plexus

As Hirschsprung's disease is related to faulty embryogenesis, it is pertinent here to consider what is known of the development of the myenteric plexus. The cyclostomes are the most primitive animals to have some sort of separate autonomic nervous system. In the lower vertebrates the vagal system is well represented, but the sympathetic system is still poorly developed (Kuntz, 1911). In embryological development the parasympathetic nerves are defined slightly before the sympathetic. Önodi (1886) studied the development of both systems and established the cerebro-spinal origin of the sympathetic trunks. He thought that the cells at the distal ends were forced to advance by the pressure of new cells behind them. However the peripheral plexuses, having no cellular connection with the cord, must have arisen *in situ*. Kohn (1907) believed that the primordia of the sympathetic trunks arose as cell columns along the aorta and did not come from the neuraxis, and that the myenteric neurones were formed in the gut. A similar view was expressed much earlier by Remak (1847). Froriep (1907) considered that cells from the neuraxis advanced along the ventral nerve roots to enter the sympathetic trunks.

Kuntz (1910) and Abel (1910, 1912) thought that the peripheral parasympathetic plexuses were derived from neurones which migrated down the vagal trunks from the medulla. Abel, working with the chick, considered that the cells were derived from the vagal and possibly the glossopharyngeal ganglia, and accompanied the vagal fibres to the gut wall. Kuntz (1910) found the same thing in mammals. He said that 12 mm embryos still had neurones visible along the vagal trunks, but at 16 mm they had gone. Tello (1924), again in the chick, found the first evidence of neurones in the myenteric plexus at 72 hours, and that differentiation proceeded rapidly during the fourth day. Van Campenhout (1932), doing grafting experiments on the chick, found that enteric grafts at 72 hours developed ganglia. At 72 hours in the chick the vagal fibres have not reached the stomach. He thought that the autonomic neurones arose from the neural crest as had been postulated by Marcus (1909). In human embryos Kuntz (1920) found that the vagus contained cells of neural origin which could be shown in direct continuity with the hind-brain and they could also be seen in abundance at the distal end of the nerve. Jones (1942) demonstrated in chick embryos, that if the hind-brain is removed at approximately the 42nd hour of incubation, the peripheral vagal ganglia fail to appear.

There has been disagreement about the origin of the intrinsic nerve cells of the colon. Jones (1942) removed the caudal portion of the neural tube at 48 hours incubation in the chick, and said that the ganglia in the colon failed to appear. Kuntz (1952) also described cells of neural origin migrating distally along the sacral nerves. He said that they were 'indifferent' cells which could differentiate into either neurones or glia and often could not be recognised until they reached the ganglia. Yntema and Hammond (1953, 1954) also did excision experiments of the neural crest and neural tube in developing chicks. They are definite that there are neurones in the wall of the intestine between 35 and 72 hours incubation before the vagal fibres arrive. If the vagal crest is removed early there are no intrinsic ganglia in the lungs, heart, oesophagus, stomach or intestine. If the vagal crest is incompletely removed there may be neurones in the anterior part of the gut and not in the posterior. Removal of the crest in the lumbosacral region had no effect on the enteric neurones as these authors say that they all come from the vagal crest. More recently Okamoto and Ueda (1967) have made a further study of the problem in human embryos. They found that at 5 weeks' gestation vagal trunks are present in the upper oesophagus and fine fibres from the pelvic nerves are seen in the rectum. There are no intramural ganglia in the alimentary tract. During the sixth week there are neuroblasts present around and along the circular muscle layer in relation to pre-existing vagal nerves. They extend only down to the cardia. By the seventh week there are neuroblasts in the oesophagus, stomach and duodenum and most of the cephalic limb of the mid-gut. By the eighth week they are present throughout the alimentary tract except the distal half of the colon and rectum. By the twelfth week there are neurones throughout the gut. After the neurones are in position the outer muscle coat is laid down outside it.

Some continued maturation of the plexus continues up to and probably after birth. Stöhr (1949) considered that there were many immature neurones in the myenteric plexus which could develop if needed. Gabella (1967) found that in the rat the density of neurones was higher in the adult.

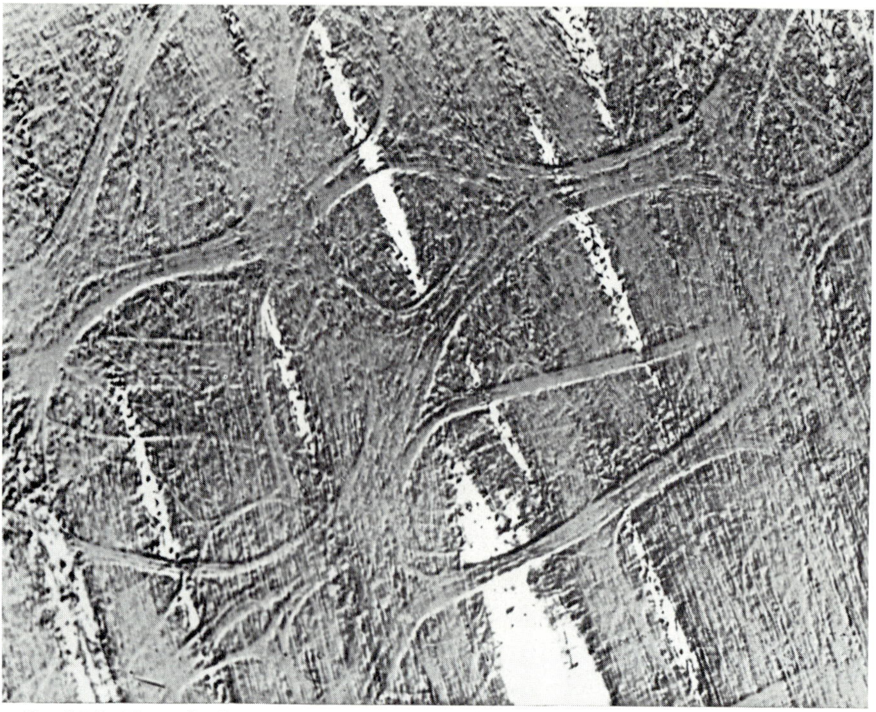

Fig. 14.4. The colonic myenteric plexus from an infant of 24 weeks' gestation. There are no argyrophil neurones to be seen at this age, and even at full-term there are only a few visible. The picture has been obtained by superimposing a positive and a negative and rephotographing.

At birth there were about 7 times the adult number in a unit area. However the increase in intestinal area with growth was about 28-fold, therefore there was a four-fold increase in visible neurones. He interprets this as due to the fact that many are undifferentiated and unidentifiable at birth. In man Blanca-Smith (1951) showed maturation of neurones in late foetal life; however Aldridge and Campbell (1968) could find no difference in the appearances between premature and full-term infants. It is possible that immature cells persist into adult life, as Storsteen *et al.* (1953) found a twofold increase in the number of ganglion cells in patients with ulcerative colitis. If this is so the most likely explanation is that the disease process has stimulated the differentiation of cells which are not normally recognisable.

In the premature infant of about 30 weeks' gestation there are nuclei in the plexus region, but it is very difficult to say whether they are ganglion cells or schwann cells (Fig. 14.4). There are usually a few definite neuronal nuclei, one or two of which have cytoplasm. On the silver preparations the small-meshed plexus is readily seen but only a small proportion of the axons are morphologically discrete. The neurones are represented by black amorphous blobs without processes and it is obvious that the proportion of argyrophil cells is lower than in the adult. During the last 10 weeks of foetal life the number of neurones indentifiable on paraffin section increases and the silver preparations show better morphology. Even at full-term, there appears to be a relative shortage of fully-developed adult neurones. It is probable that they are represented in the ganglia by a primitive type of cell which can mature into a normal neurone.

(i) The pathogenesis of Hirschsprung's disease

The evidence suggests that the myenteric neurones migrate to the wall of the distal colon possibly either along the vagus or along the parasympathetic nerves. In Hirschsprung's disease this migration fails to reach the gut to a varying degree. It could be only a partial failure, the neurones arresting somewhere along the course of the nerve, or a complete failure, in which case the migration never started. If Yntema and Hammond (1952, 1954) are correct and all the vagal neurones come from the vagal crest, the assumption must be that the process is never completed. This would fit in with the finding that it is always the most distal part of the gut which is affected, there is never a skip lesion, and the site of the upper end of the pathological area is somewhat variable.

The unmyelinated nerve trunks seen in Hirschsprung's disease are strongly cholinergic (Niemi *et al.*, 1961). They most probably represent the original vagal or possibly sacral parasympathetic outgrowth, which because the nerve cells have not arrived has not disappeared. Other possibilities are that they are processes of neurones which have not arrived, or that they are an additional supply which has grown in because the original innervation is missing. Examination of the junctional zone and the dilated segment in Hirschsprung's disease suggests that the original parasympathetic outgrowth breaks up and disappears as the neurones arrive, only a few fibres persisting as the adult extrinsic parasympathetic supply. Processes of the intrinsic neurones mingle with these trunks as part of the mature plexus. In Hirschsprung's disease this process is arrested at various stages, producing the appearances described above.

15 Toxic damage to the myenteric plexus

Many of the powerful drugs which are in use today, particularly antineoplastic agents, are neurotoxic. They give comparatively little clinical trouble because, in most instances, they do not cross the blood–brain barrier in sufficient concentration to affect central neurones. However the cells of the posterior root ganglia and the autonomic ganglia are not so protected and considerable damage may occur. If a toxin affects one particular type of cell, leaving the surrounding tissues intact, it is probably because it impairs some structure or metabolic activity which is peculiar to or predominant in that cell. For example the myenteric neurones are strongly cholinergic, and therefore are affected by anticholinergic agents; they manufacture RNA and are susceptible to drugs disrupting nucleic acid metabolism; they contain neurotubules and are damaged by agents destroying these structures and the neurone seems to be unduly dependent on pyridoxal, although this may also reflect the latter's function in nucleic acid metabolism.

(a) Atropine

Atropine is the best known of all anticholinergic agents. In the days when atropine was the only treatment available for Parkinsonism, patients were kept on daily doses for a very long time. These patients not only developed intractable constipation but at post-mortem the colon was found to be enormously dilated and thickened (Siegmund, 1935).

Twenty mice weighing between 20 and 25 g were given 0·0066 mg of atropine intraperitoneally daily for a fortnight and then left for 2–8 weeks before being killed. At death the animals were all extremely constipated with 4–8 pellets in the distal colon. In the normal mouse the myenteric plexus contains only an occasional argyrophil cell with a rather small thin body and multiple processes (Fig. 2·1), In the animals given atropine the plexus contained a large number of dark swollen cells (Plate II.2). In the most severely affected mice there were one or two fragmented axons.

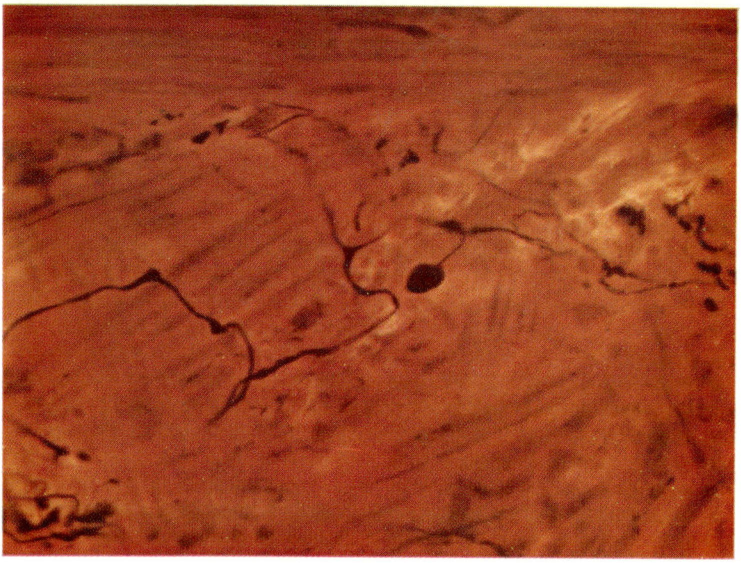

Plate II.1. The myenteric plexus from the proximal dilated segment of colon of a patient with Hirschsprung's disease. The anatomy of the innervation is grossly disturbed although neurones are present in the near neighbourhood of this field. Since the axons do not follow the normal route from one ganglion to another, normal coordinated movement cannot occur, showing that the dilated segment as well as the contracted segment is faulty in this condition.

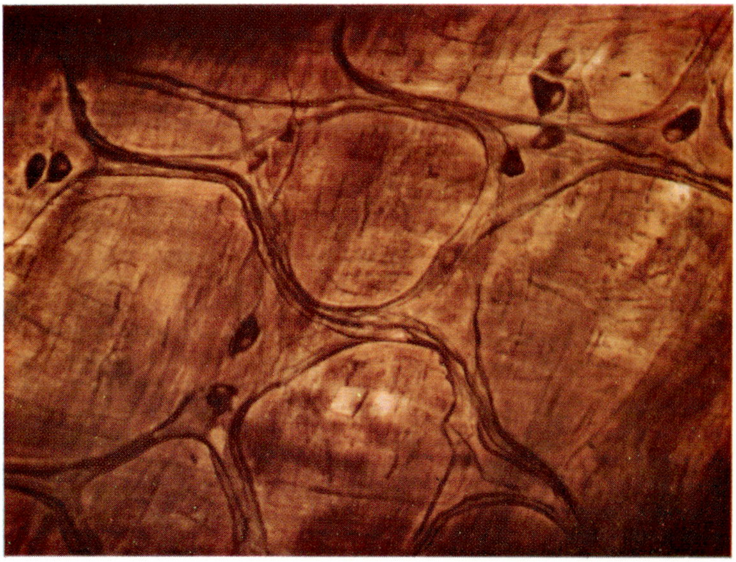

Plate II.2. The colonic myenteric plexus from a mouse, which had been given 0·006 mg atropine for 2 weeks and killed 3 days later. The neurones are swollen, globular and argyrophil (cf. Fig. 2.1, p. 7).

suggesting that the cell had died. An interesting point about these histological changes is that atropine is a simple substance with no pharmacological action of its own (Brodie, 1965). Its structure is sufficiently like that of acetylcholine to deceive the receptor at the parasympathetic nerve ending. Atropine is taken up and acetylcholine is crowded out. The complex of the receptor with atropine does not elicit a biological response. This blocking action appears to be sufficient to put the cell out of action for at least 8 weeks and to produce histological changes.

Acetylcholine is contained in synaptic vesicles at the nerve ending. It is probable but not certain that it is manufactured in the perikaryon and passes down the axon to the synapse. The amount of acetylcholine produced must be controlled by some feedback mechanism from the receptor organ. If no acetylcholine can gain access to the receptor site, the vesicles could accumulate at the ending, but more probably it is secreted normally and immediately broken down by cholinesterase. The unstimulated receptor will then demand more acetylcholine and the stress on the cell caused by gross overproduction of the transmitter could result in swelling and darkening of the perikaryon. Presumably if this stress is continued the production of acetylcholine may cease altogether.

(b) Chlorpromazine

Therapeutic substances in common use, many of which have anticholinergic properties, are the tranquillisers. It is well known that patients taking chlorpromazine in large doses suffer intractable constipation. Zimmerman (1962), while investigating another effect of the drug, noticed that when given to rats intraperitoneally it produces a megacolon, although he did not postulate a mechanism.

Chlorpromazine was given to mice weighing 20–25 g in doses of 1 mg intraperitoneally twice weekly. This dose makes them sleepy, although they are not in coma and will move when stimulated. The animals were quite alert by the next morning and there was no spontaneous mortality. Twenty animals were given 20 doses and killed within a week of the last dose. In addition 3 further animals were left for 4 months after the last does before being killed.

All the animals were extremely constipated post-mortem including those left without treatment for 4 months. Some mice had their entire distal colon packed with faeces so that it was not possible to distinguish individual pellets. Histologically the myenteric plexus showed two types of lesion. One was the presence of enlarged argyrophil neurones similar to those seen in mice treated with atropine, but there were many more fragmented axons and the changes were more severe. The other was the great increase in stainable nerve fibres within the ganglia. In some cases the ganglion was completely replaced by a tangled mass of axons (Fig. 15.1).

Chlorpromazine has at least two pharmacological actions, it is both a cholinergic and an alpha-adrenergic blocking agent. It is likely that the swollen argyrophil neurons are the result of its anticholinergic activity as is also the functional impairment. The tangles of nerve fibres are similar to those which can be produced by other adrenergic blocking agents such

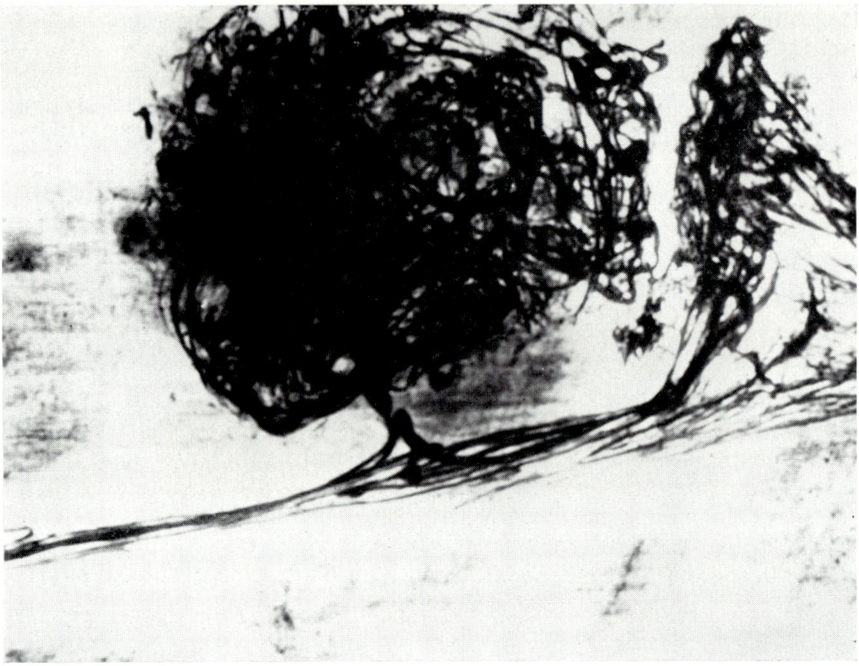

Fig. 15.1. The colonic myenteric plexus from a mouse, which had been given 1 mg of chlorpromazine twice weekly for 10 weeks. It shown an enormous overgrowth of the autonomic ground plexus. These changes are similar to those produced by other alpha adrenergic blocking agents.

as guanethidine and bretyllium (Smith, unpublished). These latter substances given to mice produce impressive histological changes but as far as can be seen no functional abnormality. The tangle of nerves must represent either gross hypertrophy of the autonomic ground plexus which is normally beyond the resolution of the light microscope or else actual growth of nerve-endings. It seems very likely that the affected fibres are the sympathetic ones which form the perineuronal networks. They have grown or hypertrophied because their transmitter has been blocked and they are endeavouring to produce more. The sympathetic innervation is comparatively unimportant in gut motility and there is no functional change. Irreversible damage to neurones in the central nervous system also occurs in patients given this drug (Ayd, 1961; Hunter *et al.*, 1964).

(c) The vinca alkaloids

Vinblastine and vincristine are used in the treatment of malignant disease, particularly the lymphomas. They impair mitosis by damaging the spindle in a similar fashion to colchicum. Patients taking the drug may develop

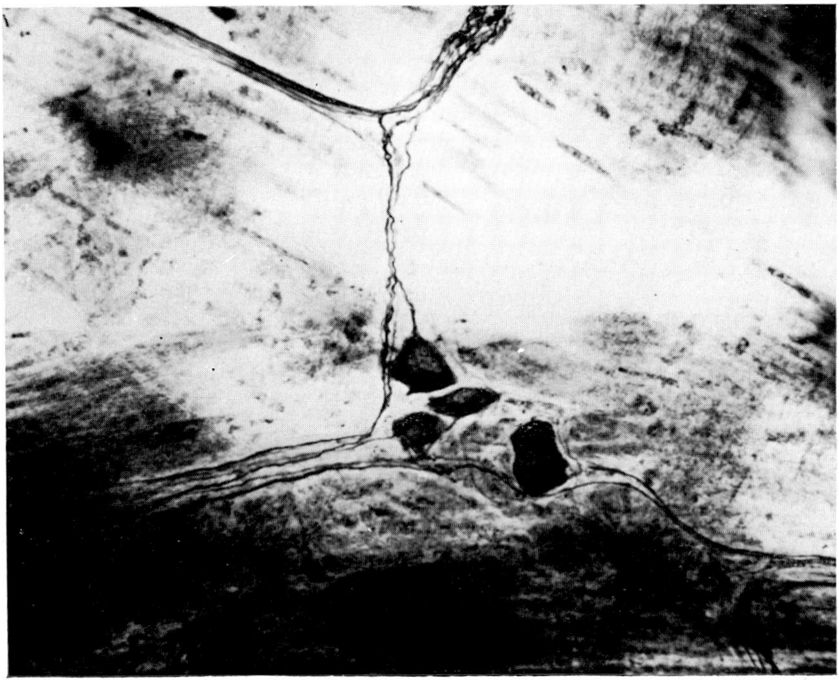

Fig. 15.2. The colonic myenteric plexus from a mouse which had received 3 doses of 0·005 mg of vinblastine sulphate. The neurones are swollen and densely argyrophil. A similar change can be produced in the neurones of the central nervous system by this drug due to the effect on the neurotubules.

considerable abdominal distension, which is mainly due to dilatation of the colon, but the small intestine is also involved. In one reported case a patient was admitted to another hospital and underwent laparotomy (Bleehen and Jelliffe, 1965). Out of 8 patients given vinblastine for choriocarcinoma, 1 developed urinary retention, 1 pain and tenderness in the parotids, 2 sinus tachycardia and 1 had an abnormal electrocardiogram

(Hertz *et al.*, 1960). Tendon reflexes are lost in the experimental animal as well as in the patient (Tobin and Sandler, 1966). These are the findings of an extensive neuropathy involving autonomic neurones and root ganglia neurones, that is, all those not protected by the blood–brain barrier. The damage is probably due to the effect of the drug on neurotubules, which is similar in nature to that on spindle tubules (Wisneiwski *et al.*, 1968). Ultrastructural studies have been done in man and animals on the neurones affected by the drug (Shelanski and Wisniewski, 1969). The neurotubules

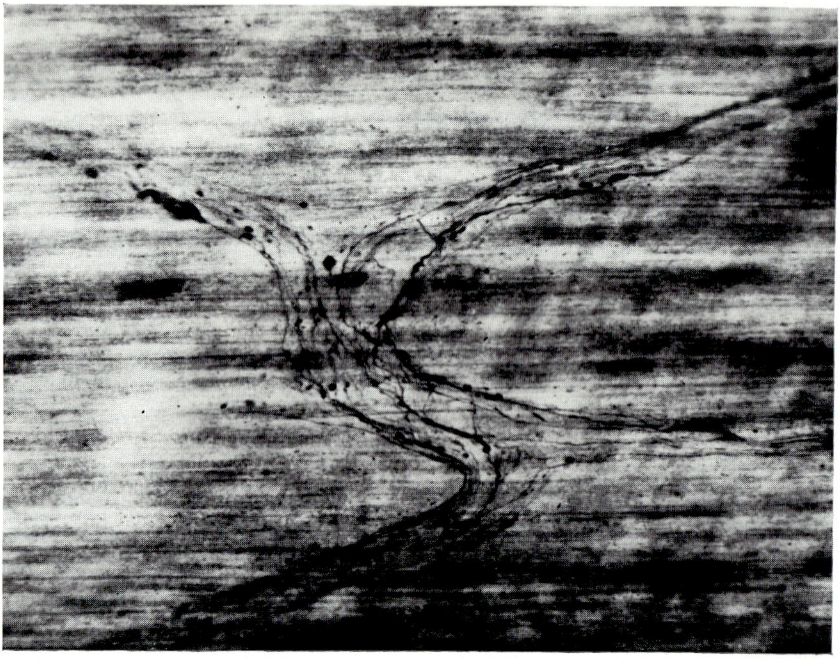

Fig. 15.3. The colonic myenteric plexus from a mouse which had received 3 doses of 0·005 mg of vinblastine sulphate. The axons are studied with argyrophil swellings (cf. Fig. 2.2).

are converted into neurofilaments producing a neurofibrillary change similar to that seen in Alzheimer's disease. The value of the blood–brain barrier as a protection is well exemplified by a case in which extensive damage to the central nervous system was produced by giving it intrathecally (Schochet *et al.*, 1968).

Used experimentally these substances are very toxic. Vinblastine sulphate was given intraperitoneally to mice in doses of either 0·05 or 0·005 mg daily (Smith, 1967*c*). Six doses were as much as they would tolerate even of the smaller amount. Out of 30 injected only 18 survived to come to post-mortem. These showed considerable dilatation of the proximal colon and distal ileum which were full of soft faecal material. The distal colon was packed with hard faeces.

Histologically the myenteric plexus showed very extensive damage. There was argyrophilia and swelling of neurones. Some of the cells were jet black but it was not possible to make out neurofibrillary change (Fig. 15.2). The neuronal processes were bulbous and irregular and there was plexus

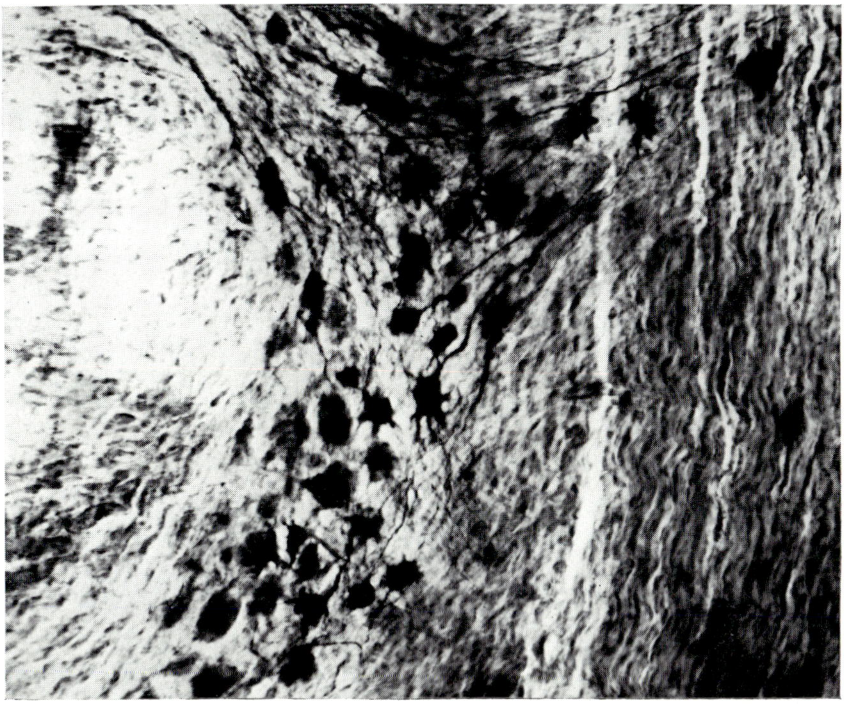

Fig. 15.4. A colonic myenteric ganglion from a patient who had been under treatment with vincristine. There are more argyrophil cells than normal because some of the argyrophobe cells have stained up. This is due to the effect of the drug on the neurotubules. At this stage the damage is probably reversible.

disintegration with retraction balls (Fig. 15.3). The changes were severe and at this dose irreversible.

The colon was examined from post-mortems of 8 patients who had been treated with vincristine, 2 of whom had developed considerable intestinal dilation, mainly of the large intestine. In these cases the important histological change was immediately apparent under low magnification. There were far too many argyrophil cells (Fig. 15.4). When the ganglia were examined under high power it was noted that the argyrophil cells were very dark but otherwise normal, and many more lightly argyrophil cells were present. These were rounded with an indistinct cell margin and no visible processes. These presumably were the argyrophobe cells which the increase in neurofilaments had rendered visible. In the patients there was no evidence of plexus break-up, and at this dosage the lesion is reversible.

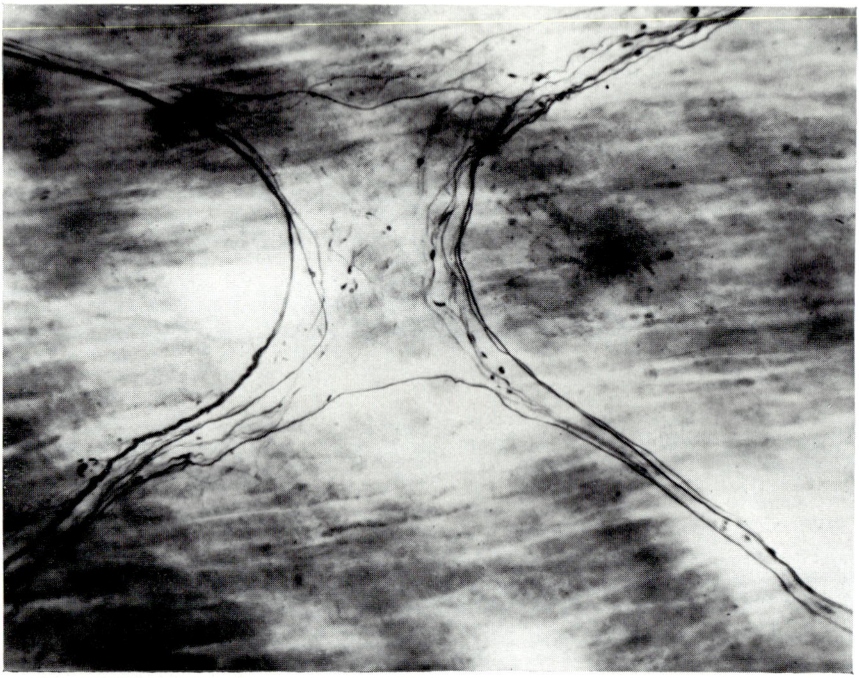

Fig. 15.5. The colonic myenteric plexus from a mouse which had been given 3 mg of mepacrine methane sulphonate daily for 5 days and killed 3 days later. There are a number of axonal and dendritic swellings (cf. Fig. 2.2, p. 8).

(d) Mepacrine

In 1966 Keeler *et al.* gave mepacrine intraperitoneally to rats and produced an enteromegaly. They showed that after 5 consecutive daily doses of 10 mg of quinacrine the animals became sick and yellow, and 1–3 weeks later abdominal distension appeared. Pathologically there was considerable dilatation of the proximal colon and distal ileum, the distal colon appearing normal. The gut wall was considerably thickened so the condition was a true enteromegaly. Histologically the muscle coats showed hypertrophy and hyperplasia and mitotic figures were seen. The authors showed that these animals had steatorrhoea. The intestinal transit time using a faecal marker was 10–16 hours in the normal rats and 24–48 hours in the quinacrine-treated rats. In their preparations which were transverse paraffin sections the ganglion cells in Auerbach's plexus were normal. In spite of this statement all the other findings in this paper strongly suggested there was a plexus lesion including the bowel wall hypertrophy, the steatorrhoea and the increased transit time.

In order to demonstrate an affinity of mepacrine for neurones, a group

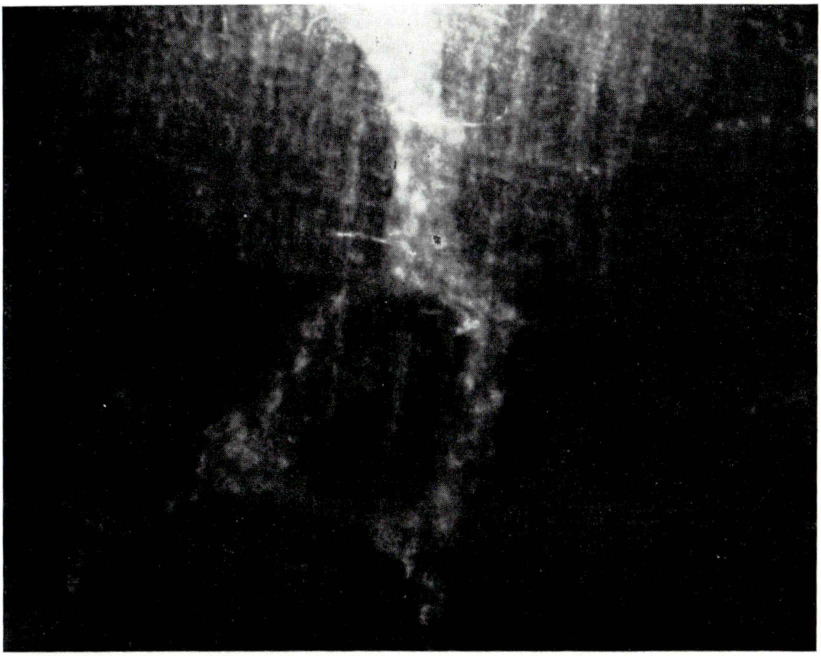

Fig. 15.6. The colonic myenteric plexus from a mouse given mepacrine methane sulphonate intraperitoneally and killed 20 minutes later. The neurones have taken up the drug and are fluorescent when viewed by ultra-violet light. This suggests that this substance has a specific affinity to nucleic acids particularly RNA.

of 6 animals were given 10 mg of mepacrine methane sulphonate intraperitoneally and killed 20 minutes later. The mucosa was removed and the gut examined under the fluorescent microscope. The drug had localised to the neurones which showed a bright yellow fluorescence (Fig. 15.6). A further group of animals were given the same drug 3 mg intraperitoneally for 5 days and killed a week later (Smith, 1967*c*). They did not thrive on this regime but they did not become yellow or seriously ill, although some developed abdominal distension. When the drug was stopped they recovered quickly. At post-mortem the caecum and proximal colon were somewhat dilated and usually contained no faeces, but only a quantity of evil-smelling fluid. Histologically paraffin sections of the colon were normal. The silver preparations showed a large number of axonal and dendritic swellings mainly in the ganglis (Fig. 15.5) and in a few animals there was some disruption of the plexus.

These findings suggest that mepacrine has an affinity for the myenteric neurones. Its initial action is a purgative one but when the dose was repeated it produced histological damage and paralysis with gut dilatation. The fact that the colon was usually empty might indicate an effect on the small intestine as well, emptying most of its contents first and later impairing peristalsis. This would be supported by the fact that Keeler *et al.* (1966) noted an increase in transit time after 5 days' treatment. The malabsorption which their animals showed is seen in man when the myenteric plexus is damaged in the small intestine, but it is interesting that it could come on so quickly. The lack of peristalsis should not be a factor because segmentation, which is mainly responsible for mixing and presenting a varying aspect of the bolus to the villi, is increased. The lengthened transit time should also help absorption. The most likely explanation is the increase in bacterial flora, a type of 'blind-loop syndrome', which occurs in the absence of small gut peristalsis.

Mepacrine is one of the acridines, which are antimitotic and antibacterial substances. They have been shown to attach themselves between the two layers of the base pairs of the DNA molecule (Albert, 1965). As these layers are normally almost touching, the DNA helix becomes extended by this intercalation. The extension is accomplished by a slight unwinding of the molecule without any rupture of the hydrogen bonds. X-ray diffraction patterns (Lerman, 1961) showed that although the meridional spacing of 3–4 10^{-1} nm was retained, there was a decrease in the mass per unit length. The effect of this on function is that although DNA synthesis is not impaired the production of RNA ceases because the template is damaged. As discussed above neurones make a large amount of RNA and this could be the basis of the toxic effect. However these tricyclic compounds are very active and it could be due to some other factor.

(e) Daunorubicin

Daunorubicin is used in the treatment of leukaemia, particularly the acute myeloblastic type. It is antineoplastic because of its effect on nucleic acid metabolism. It complexes with DNA (Calendi *et al.*, 1965) and probably intercalates with the molecule as do the acridines (Goldberg, 1965). It is very toxic, causing marrow aplasia and cardiac abnormalities which occasionally result in cardiac failure. In association with cardiac muscle damage there is evidence of changes in the intrinsic cardiac neurones

(Smith, 1969). Clinical evidence suggests that the drug is concentrated in the heart and in human material the myenteric neurones show only minor changes, in contrast to those of the heart itself. However if the drug is given intraperitoneally to mice, thus putting it in very close proximity to the myenteric neurones, the damage to the plexus is devastating. Mice, 20–25 g in weight, were given doses of 5 mg to the kilogram twice weekly

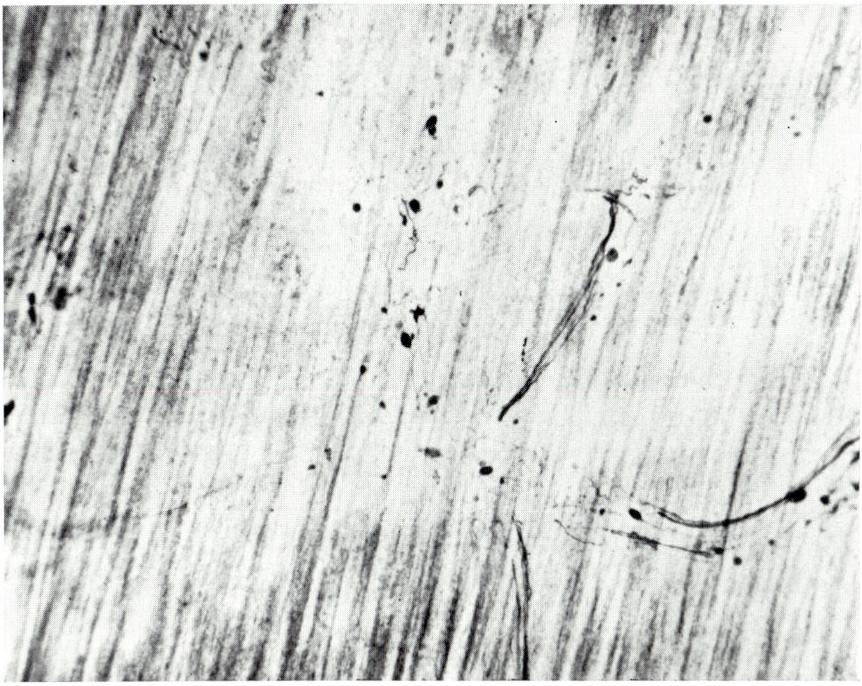

Fig. 15.7. The colonic myenteric plexus of a mouse which had been given 5 doses of daunorubicin, 10 mg to the kg. The plexus is fragmented and many axons completely disrupted. It probably causes the damage by complexing with DNA and preventing RNA synthesis (cf. Fig. 2.2, p. 8).

for 6 doses. They became ill, with 'staring' fur but no evidence of paralysis. At post-mortem they were constipated with some dilatation of the proximal colon. Histology showed axonal and dendritic swellings with in places complete fragmentation of the plexus (Fig. 15.7).

(f) Isonicotinic acid hydrazide (INH)

INH is known to be neurotoxic both in man and in animals. In man it can produce fits given in very large doses and occasional cases have been seen in which dementia has occurred after very prolonged therapy. However although it must cross the blood–brain barrier it normally does so in relatively small quantities. The much commoner complication of INH therapy is peripheral neuropathy, the 'burning feet syndrome'. This can be prevented by the simultaneous administration of pyridoxine.

INH has been used by a number of authors to produce peripheral neuropathy in the experimental animal, usually in rather large doses (Klinghardt, 1954; Cavanagh, 1967). This neuropathy can be prevented

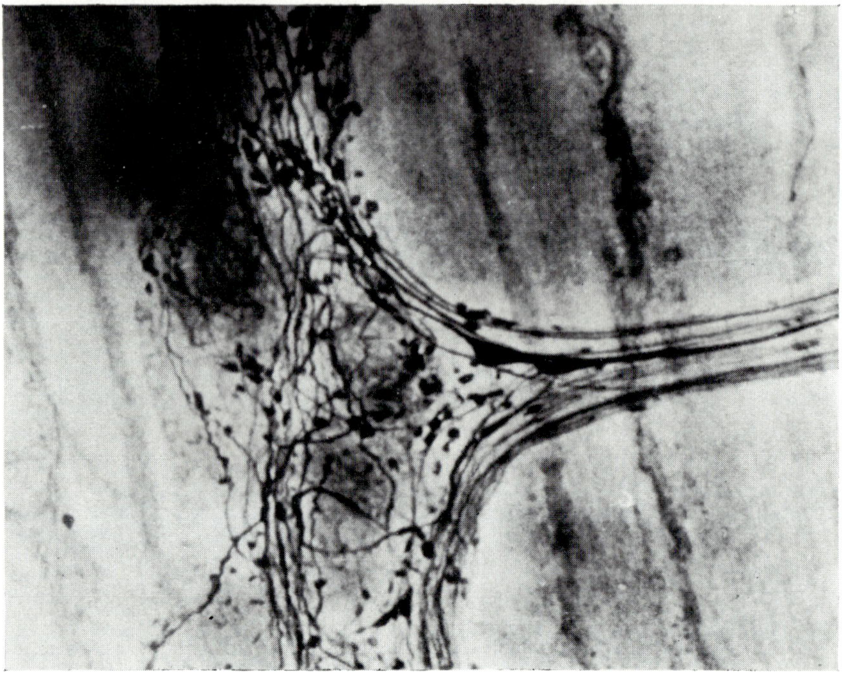

Fig. 15.8. The colonic myenteric plexus from a mouse which had received INH 5 mg intreperitoneally twice weekly for 20 doses. There is gross disorganisation of the ganglion with numerous axonal and dendritic swellings.

by giving pyridoxine (Zbinden and Stüder, 1955). Pyridoxine deficiency alone without the administration of INH may produce changes in cortical neurones (Victor and Adams, 1956).

INH was given to 12 mice weighing between 20 and 25 g in doses of 5 mg twice weekly for up to 20 doses (Smith, 1967*c*). This produced damage to posterior root ganglia neurones in addition to changes in the myenteric plexus. These consisted of a large number of neuronal and dendritic swellings similar to those seen in animals given mepacrine (Fig. 15.8). The damage to the plexus was very extensive.

The mechanism of the neuronal damage produced by the drug could be due to derangement of any of the metabolic systems that are pyridoxine-dependent. A likely possibility is the one-carbon transfer system important for nucleic acid synthesis. An animal rendered pyridoxine-deficient will accept a skin-graft which is rejected as soon as pyridoxine is added to the diet (Stoerk and Eisen, 1946; Axelrod and Trakatellis, 1964). These latter authors went on to show that this immunological failure was due to impaired RNA synthesis. Tumor grafts also do not take in the pyridoxine-deficient animal (Mihich and Nichol, 1959). It is therefore possible that the neuronal damage produced by INH is due to impaired RNA synthesis.

(g) Conclusion

These findings suggest that the myenteric plexus is unduly exposed to the action of neurotoxic drugs compared with the central nervous system. Many patients, therefore, particularly those on tranquillisers, might be expected to suffer from organic constipation. Occasionally there is acute dysfunction and deaths have been reported from paralytic ileus in patients given amitryptiline (Burkitt and Sutcliffe, 1961; Gander and Devlin, 1963).

There appear to be three types of histological damage produced by these toxins, which are distinguishable at light microscopic level. The first is produced by anticholinergic agents and affects mainly the colon although the cardia may be involved. The histological change associated with this consists of dark, swollen neurones, with, in severe cases, some axonal break-up. The second is probably produced by substances which affect nucleic acid metabolism. It is associated initially with purgation but the neurones quickly succumb, and this is followed by gut dilatation and constipation. The histological changes consist of large numbers of axonal and dendritic swellings. These changes are also seen in animals given irritant purgatives (p. 98) which might indicate a similar type of mechanism. The third type of change is produced by substances which damage neurotubules. The cells darken from an increase in neurofibrils and are eventually destroyed.

16 Cathartic colon

Purgatives of one type or another are some of the most widely used of all drugs. A type of folklore exists which teaches that the colon is a sink of iniquity which needs clearing out at frequent intervals. It is not at all uncommon for parents to give their perfectly normal children a dose of salts every Saturday night and a number of people take proprietary preparations containing cascara sagrada or senna before going to bed. This idea is not confined to the lay public. Ward sisters are notorious for purging their patients, usually without medical supervision. Travell (1954) has calculated that in one 1200-bedded hospital in New York, 406,942 doses of purgatives were given in one year, of which 127,000 were cascara or senna. This adds up to about a fifth of a ton of irritant purgatives. The greatest exploiters of this obsession are the patent medicine vendors, but the medical profession has also made its profits. Arbuthnot Lane removed a large number of colons for no very good reason and considerable financial gain to himself. His mortality rate was 28%.

Among the large number of people who take purgatives regularly there is a small group who become addicts and psychologically dependent on them. They seem to suffer from two different syndromes. Far the commonest is that of increasingly intractable constipation and they take larger and larger doses with less and less effect. In a few cases they suffer not from constipation but diarrhoea and it tends to be this group which get potassium deficiency with muscular weakness and electrocardiographic abnormalities (Schwartz and Relman, 1953; Aitchison, 1958; Houghton and Pears, 1958). A feature of this type of addiction is that patients frequently deny that they are taking laxatives which are smuggled into hospital to them by their relatives. This makes for diagnostic difficulties and if the cause of the condition is appreciated and the purgatives withdrawn, it may precipitate psychiatric disturbances.

A typical clinical history of this type of condition was given by Avery Jones (1967). She was a woman of 52, who complained of increasing constipation since a child. When she was 26, she was operated on for anal fissure. She took aperients frequently and had attacks of pain and a feeling of abdominal distension. In 1961 at the age of 46, she had a sigmoid loop resected without effect on her symptoms, and a year later an operation for anal stenosis. She was having three or four fluid stools a day and was very tired, presumably due to potassium deficiency. She finally had a total colectomy with improvement in her symptoms. It is common in this condition for patients to have a succession of less radical procedures before coming to colectomy.

The reason why there should be two different syndromes is not clear, but it may be simply related to the amount of various types of purgatives

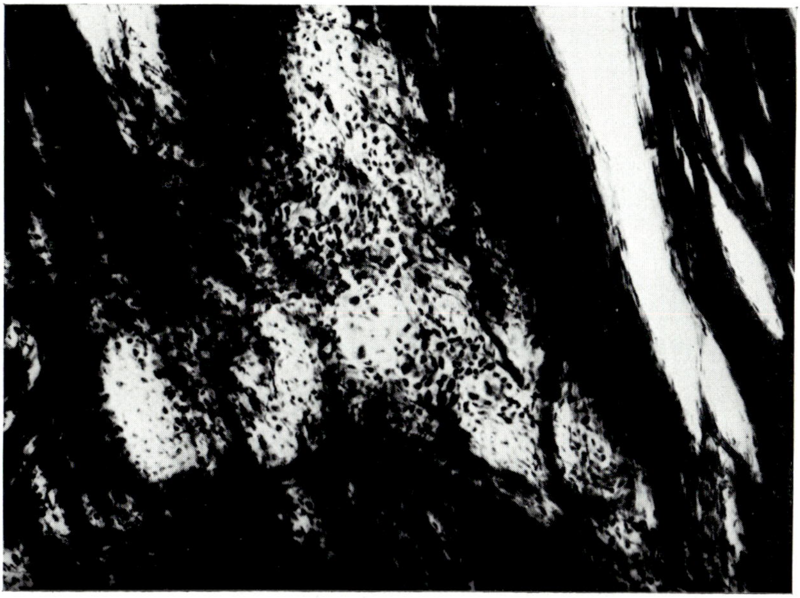

Fig. 16.1. A ganglion from the sigmoid colon of a purgative addict of 63. He had been taking laxatives for about 40 years. The ganglion contains no argyrophil cells, but a few nuclei of non-argyrophil cells can be seen in the centre. The appearance of the paraffin section were normal apart from the melanosis coli.

taken. It is almost impossible to obtain a detailed account from a purgative addict of what drugs they have been taking, and in what quantity. Many proprietary preparations contain two or more substances in the same tablet and in addition this type of patient frequently changes his tablets in search of better ones. If, for example, he had been taking a great deal of phenolphthalein together with the anthraquinone, the overall effect might be different to that following the latter drug alone. Animal experiments suggest that senna alone probably produces intractable constipation (p. 98). Until we know more about the pharmacology of all types of purgatives we cannot answer this problem.

The pathology of the colon in the purgative addict shows three changes. There is marked thinning of the muscle coat with considerable dilatation, and very little haustration. The transverse colon is often pendulous and the sigmoid very large on barium enema. This thinning of the bowel wall helps to distinguish the condition from organic constipation due to other causes of plexus damage in which the bowel wall is thickened. There is melanosis coli, more striking on the right side than the left. In this condition the mucosa appears black, either in patches or as a continuous

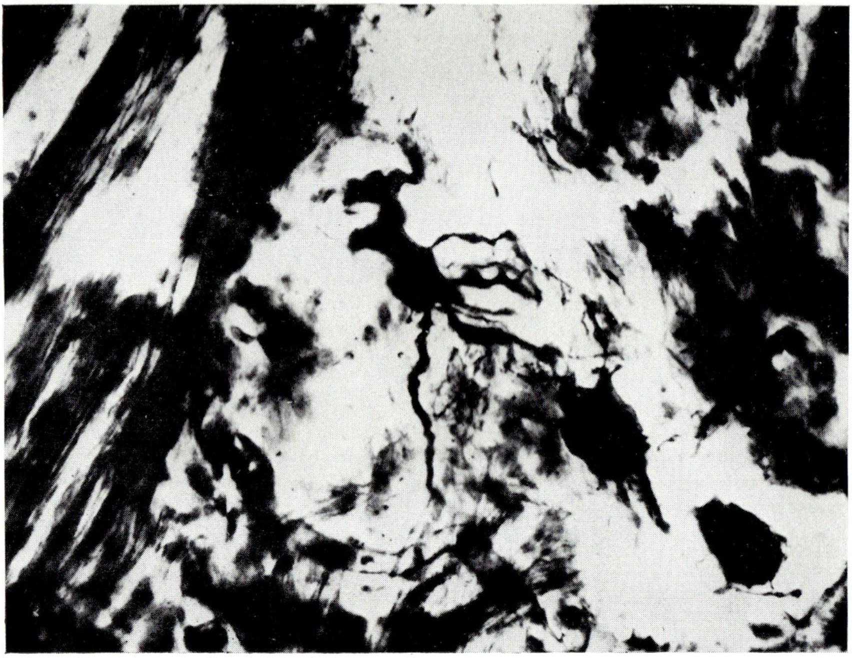

Fig. 16.2. A ganglion from the colon of a man who had been taking cathartics in large doses for about 30 years. The neurones are very dark, shrunken and distorted with irregular processes.

sheet. This is due to collections of pigment-containing macrophages in the mucosa. The pigment is not melanin, but its chemistry has not been identified. It contains some lipid and it has been thought by some to be a wear-and-tear pigment. Thirdly there is extensive damage to the myenteric plexus itself. This damage is also worse on the right side of the colon than the left. In very long-standing cases, usually 30–40 years, it consists of a loss of argyrophil neurones with an increase of schwann cells (Fig. 16.1). The remaining neurones are dark and shrunken, with clubbed or swollen processes (Fig. 16.2). In two patients, one male and one female, who had a colectomy for cathartic colon under the age of 30, the history of purgative addiction, although severe, was necessarily shorter. In these cases there was also some loss of neurones with schwannosis but some of the remaining cells were pale and enormously swollen (Fig. 16.3). The dark shrunken cells were not seen. This might suggest that the purgatives produce an initial over-stimulation before they destroy. In the cases of cathartic

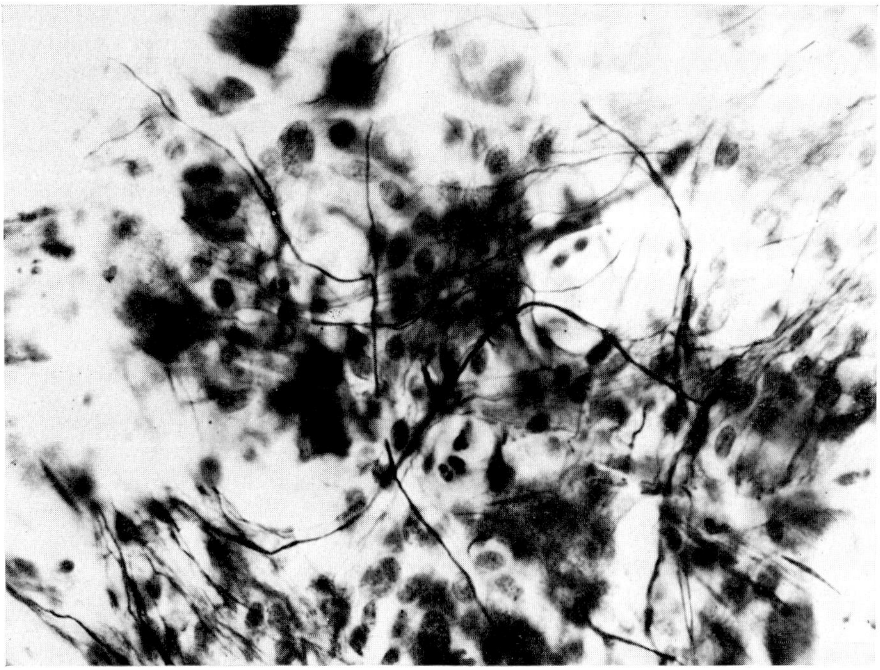

Fig. 16.3. A ganglion cell from the ascending colon removed from a purgative addict aged 29. As this patient was still young she cannot have been taking laxatives for many years. In this case the loss of neurones was not very severe but the remaining ones were grossly swollen and rather pale, although the processes were probably normal. This may represent a state of over-stimulation of the ganglion cell occurring early in the condition. In the ensuing years these cells will die. (cf. Fig. 16.2 same magnification).

colon coming to colectomy, the fall-out is severe, and it is unlikely that there would be any spontaneous recovery even if the purgatives were stopped.

The mode of action of some groups of purgatives is obvious, such as the osmotic group, including magnesium sulphate, and the lubricants, including liquid paraffin. Calomel acts by damaging the mucous membrane and producing a frank colitis. This was a frequent cause of death in the heyday of purgation for every known disease. However there is an important group of cathartics whose mode of action is not so clear. These are the anthraquinones or irritant purgatives, including cascara, senna and rhubarb. It is astounding that so little is known of the pharmacology of such common medicaments.

The active principles of these drugs are emodines, which are hydroxymethyl anthraquinones. Aloes emodine (1,8-dihydroxy-3-hydroxymethyl anthraquinone) is found in aloes, cascara and senna. Frangula emodine (1,6,8-trihydroxy-3-methyl anthraquinone) is found in cascara, and there are a number of similar substances found in these drugs. The pure chemical compound, dihydroxyanthraquinone, is also used in some preparations. This is considerably more expensive than the natural product and there is no evidence that it is any more effective.

There is a latent period between giving the drug and purgation of about 10 hours. It was assumed that this was the time taken for it to pass down the gut, the substance being ineffective in the small intestine but working in the large, either because it had been changed chemically during passage or because of local sensitivity. This statement is still seen in modern textbooks of pharmacology although Straub and Triendl showed in 1937 that it was absorbed in the small intestine and re-excreted into the large. They did this by feeding it by mouth to cats with a divided intestine, showing that the interval between administration and purgation was about the same as in the normal. How it produces purgation when in the colon has not been certainly demonstrated. Most writers assume with Martindale (1967) that it irritates the mucosa and that the muscular contraction is reflex. Douthwaite and Goulding (1957) gave 180 mg of sennakot to mice by stomach tube. This produced purgation in 12 hours, but repeating it daily up to 11 days produced no inflammatory change in the gut. These authors comment on the paucity of information about the mode of action of this substance. Fairbairn (1958) gave weekly doses for 9 months without ill-effect or tolerance. Okada (1940) gave senna to dogs and recorded colonic pressure changes with intraluminal balloons. He thought that they produced the same type of pressure wave as normal peristalsis. He suggested that the *Escherichia coli* converted the emodines to oxyanthraquinone and that this substance acted on Auerbach's plexus. Straub and Triendl (1937) said that the action of senna was to increase peristalsis without effect on the pendulum movements. They also noted that it impaired water absorption by the large intestine. In the same year Grabfield (1937) perfused 1/10,000 cascara sagrada through the isolated intestine. He said that it increased peristalsis in the large intestine, but was without effect on the small. After peristalsis was established in the colon there was some increase in activity of the small intestine, which he said was reflex.

The pure substances anthracene and anthraquinone, if given parenterally, are lethal in extremely small doses, so that it is impossible to use them for experimental purposes. When anthraquinone is given intravenously, the animal dies instantaneously and the heart does not continue beating, suggesting that it is a very powerful cell poison. If the substance is administered by mouth only a small amount is absorbed if it is given alone. However, the U.S. patent 2,851,394 contains the following comment:

'It was further found in our laboratory that the oral administration of 1,8 dihydroxyanthraquinone did not produce death in rats even in quantities as much as 22 mg/kg. On the other hand, when this substance was administered in combination with non-toxic amounts of dioctyl sodium

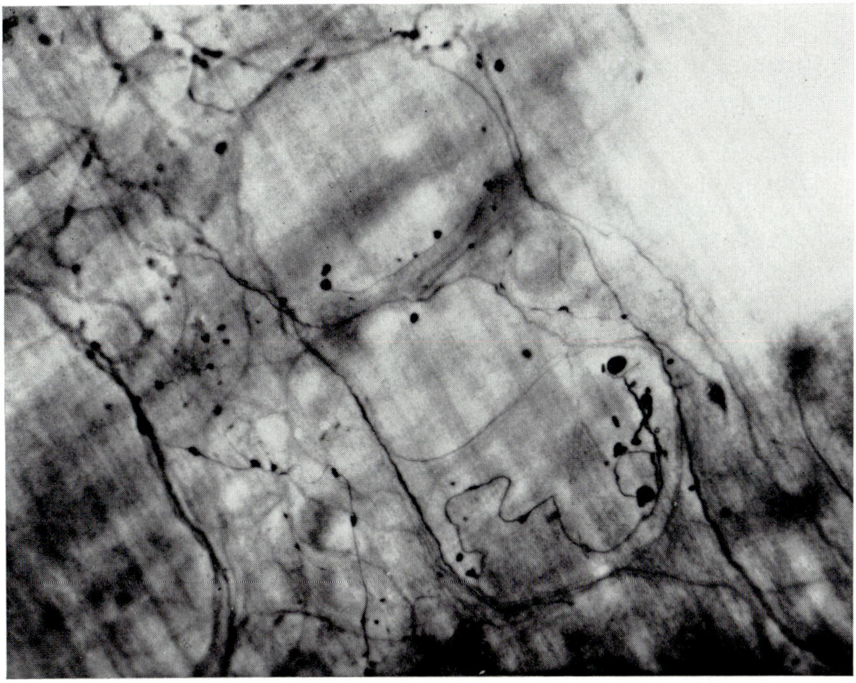

Fig. 16.4. The colonic myenteric plexus of a mouse which had received 1 ml of a 1% solution of syrup of senna intraperitoneally daily for a fortnight. A number of axonal swellings are present.

sulfosuccinate only 9 mg/kg was sufficient to give a 50% kill in rats. This effect can only be due to increased absorption since the animals die with symptoms of systemic toxicity.'

Dioctyl sodium sulfosuccinate is itself a mild laxative, but it is used by pharmacologists to increase the absorption of a number of drugs.

Syrup of senna, given intraperitoneally, is lethal in a dose of about 1 ml of a 20% solution. One millitre of a 1% solution is a mild purgative dose. If a larger dose is given the colon may be empty as far back as the ileo-caecal valve.

Two groups of experiments were done giving syrup of senna to mice (Smith, 1968). In the first, animals were given 5% syrup of senna in lieu of drinking water for a period of up to 6 months. Syrup of senna contains, in addition to the senna, a little liquorice and some sugar. The animals who drank nothing else suffered no apparent ill effects. The second group of animals were given 1 ml of a 1% solution of syrup of senna intraperitoneally daily for a fortnight. When the animals were killed the colon contained more faecal pellets than normal. In the group given the drug intraperitoneally this was more striking, the whole distal colon in some cases being packed with bulky faeculent material, which was not broken up into pellets. They therefore showed clinical evidence of motility failure.

Histologically the plexus showed a varying degree of damage, the change consisting of fragmentation of the axons with axonal and dendritic swellings (Fig. 16.4). The picture was very similar to that produced by mepacrine.

The anthraquinones have therefore been shown to produce destruction of the myenteric plexus in animals. Many neurotoxic substances will stimulate neurones in small doses. If this is the mode of action of the irritant purgatives it would account for the necessity for larger and larger doses as the neural damage increases and also for the overactive neurones seen in cases with a short history. The fact that increased absorption reduces the lethal dose so strikingly in animals and that they die of systemic toxicity suggests that it may be unwise to add substances to anthraquinones which will increase their absorption.

In man the standard preparations of the vegetable laxatives, cascara, senna and aloes, are undoubtedly safe even in enormous doses. Patients who die from purgative addiction, die from the metabolic side-effects, not anthraquinone overdosage. This safety is probably due to two factors, one is that, given by mouth, the amount of active principle absorbed is very small, and the other is that what is absorbed is concentrated in the colon. This is a good example of the fact that the way the body distributes a given drug may be more important pharmacologically than the actual biochemical effect on the cell. They do, however, if taken for long enough damage the colon. They probably do this by a direct toxic effect on the tissue in which they are concentrated—the smooth muscle and its contained plexus. It is probable that the pigment found in the mucosa is a tissue break-down product, analogous to the lipofuscin found in brown atrophy of the heart, possibly combined with the anthraquinone itself or a metabolic product therefrom. The histology of the mucosa appears normal, although no quantitative studies have been done on it. It is so close to the muscle that its function may be affected and it is known that water absorption is impaired in the cathartic.

In summary, therefore, purgative addiction lasting many years may produce so much damage to the colonic muscle and its innervation, that the only possible treatment is to remove it.

17 Conclusions

Damage to the myenteric plexus at any level in the alimentary canal results in failure of peristalsis and loss of reflexes which are dependent on an intact nerve supply. Loss of the intrinsic innervation of the gut produces marked dilatation of the lumen and hypertrophy of the smooth muscle. This dilatation and hypertrophy may in itself exacerbate the patient's symptoms.

The myenteric plexus contains two types of neurones distinguished by their affinity for silver. The argyrophil cells are few in number and their processes do not leave the plexus, terminating on other neurones, argyrophil and argyrophobe, in the same or neighbouring ganglia. The argyrophobe cells secrete acetylcholine and give branches to the muscle The argyrophil cells could be acting in a supervisory capacity and be internuncial neurones in the parasympathetic supply. Lesions of the argyrophil cells only will produce the same clinical picture as a total fall-out of cells The two types cannot be distinguished on paraffin, haematoxylin and eosin preparations, which accounts for the difficulty in diagnosing some myenteric plexus disorders.

In the oesophagus myenteric fall-out causes achalasia, with failure to relax the gastro-oesophageal segment in response to distension of the ampulla. In the stomach it results in hypertrophic pyloric stenosis, which is a failure of the pyloric pump mechanism and a reduction in the lumen of the pyloric canal from secondary muscle hypertrophy. In the small intestine, if the aperistaltic segment is long there is intermittent intestinal obstruction and malabsorption from the functional blind loop. The colon is very dependent on the myenteric plexus, because the contents are more solid, and it is probable that constipation can be produced by a lesion which would not be sufficiently severe to give symptoms elsewhere in the gut. Megacolon with intractable constipation and a dilated and thickened large bowel may be congenital or acquired.

Since the myenteric neurones are outside the blood–brain barrier, they can be easily affected by circulating neurotoxins. The anti-cholinergic drugs, particularly the tranquillisers, damage the neurones, probably the argyrophobe cells, producing severe constipation. The vinca alkaloids affect the neurotubules in the same way as they affect the spindle and large doses can produce acute gut distension with peristaltic failure. Antimitotic agents given for malignant disease with a view to disrupting nucleic acid metabolism will affect RNA-dependent neurones if they reach them in large enough concentration although this is rare in clinical practice.

Diseases of the myenteric plexus producing impairment of intestinal motility have not received the attention they deserve. They are frequently misdiagnosed and repeated ineffective laparotomies add to the patient's misfortunes. In some instances a vagotomy is done, which can hardly fail to make the condition worse. Patients with organic constipation are lost among the bowel-conscious multitudes. Patients on chlorpromazine complaining of constipation are given cascara, which is ineffective if the neurones are damaged.

In order to help these patients we need to know a great deal more about the physiology and pathology of the autonomic control of gut motility, but it is hoped that the information provided here will at least help in making a correct diagnosis.

Bibliography

ABEL, W. (1910). The development of the autonomic nervous mechanism of the alimentary canal of the bird. *Proc. roy. Soc. Edinb.* **30,** 327.

— (1912). Further observations on the development of the sympathetic nervous system in the chick. *J. Anat. (Lond.)* **47,** 35.

ADAMS, C. W. M., BRAIN, R. H. F., ELLIS, F. G., KAUNTZE, R. and TROUNCE, J. R. (1961). Achalasia of the cardia. *Guy's Hosp. Rep.* **110,** 191.

ADAMS, C. W. M., MARPLES, E. A. and TROUNCE, J. R. (1960). Achalasia of the cardia and Hirschsprung's disease. The amount and distribution of cholinesterases. *Clin. Sci.* **19,** 473.

ADAMS, H. D. (1964). Amyenteric achalasia of the esophagus. *Surg. Gynec. Obstet.* **119,** 251.

ADAMSON, W. A. D. and AIRD, I. (1932). Megacolon. Evidence in favour of a neurogenic origin. *Brit. J. Surg.* **20,** 220.

ADLER, H. F. and TEMPLETON, R. D. (1940). The correlation of activity and transportation in the colon of the dog. *Amer. J. Physiol.* **128,** 514.

ADLER, S. (1959). Darwin's illness. *Nature (Lond.)* **184,** 1102.

AGOSTONI, E., CHINNOCK, J. E., DALY, M. DE B. and MURRAY, J. G. (1957). Functional and histologic studies of the vagus nerve and its branches to the heart, lungs and abdominal viscera in the cat. *J. Physiol. (Lond.)* **135,** 182.

AITCHISON, J. D. (1958). Hypokalaemia following chronic diarrhoea from overuse of cascara and a deficient diet. *Lancet* **ii,** 75.

ALAROTU, H. (1956). The histopathologic changes in the myenteric plexus of the pylorus in hypertrophic pyloric stenosis of infants (Pylorospasm). *Acta paediat. scand.* **45,** Suppl. 107, 1.

ALAROTU, H. and CHRISTENSEN, E. (1949). Studies on changes in the sympathetic ganglia of the pyloric portion of the stomach in infants with pylorospasm. *Acta paediat. scand.* (Suppl.) **77,** 250.

ALBERT, A. (1965). *Selective Toxicity.* London: Methuen, p. 207.

ALDRIDGE, R. T. and CAMPBELL, P. E. (1968). Ganglion cell distribution in the normal rectum and anal canal. A basis for the diagnosis of Hirschsprung's disease by anorectal biopsy. *J. pediat. Surg.* **3,** 475.

ALNOR, P. (1958). On the pathogenesis of cardiospasm. An experimental study. *J. thorac. Surg.* **36,** 141.

ALVAREZ, W. C. (1940). *An Introduction to Gastro-enterology* (4th edition). New York: Hoeber, p. 382.

— (1949). A simple explanation for cardiospasm and Hirschsprung's disease. *Gastroenterology* **13,** 422.

ARMITAGE, G. and RHIND, J. A. (1951). The fate of the tumour in infantile hypertrophic pyloric stenosis. *Brit. J. Surg.* **39,** 39.

ATKINSON, M., EDWARDS, D. A. W., HONOUR, A. J. and ROWLANDS, E. N. (1957). Comparison of cardiac and pyloric sphincters, a manometric study. *Lancet* **ii,** 918.

CARTER, C. O. (1961). The inheritance of congenital pyloric stenosis. *Brit. med. Bull.* **17,** 251.

CARVETH, S. W., SCHLEGEL, J. F., CODE, C. F. and ELLIS, F. H., JR. (1960). Changes in the motor action of the esophagus and the gastroesophageal sphincter after vagotomy in dogs. *Surg. Forum* **11,** 311.

CASH, J. T. (1886). Contribution to the study of intestinal rest and movement. *Proc. roy. Soc. B* **41,** 212.

CASSELLA, R. R., BROWN, A. L., JR., SAYRE, G. P. and ELLIS, F. H., JR. (1964). Achalasia of the esophagus. Pathologic and etiologic considerations. *Ann. Surg.* **160,** 474.

CASSELLA, R. R., ELLIS, F. H., JR. and BROWN, A. L. (1965*a*). Fine-structure changes in achalasia of esophagus. 1. Vagus nerves. *Amer. J. Path.* **46,** 279.

— (1965*b*). Fine-structure changes in achalasia of esophagus. 2. Esophageal smooth muscle. *Amer. J. Path.* **46,** 467.

CAVANAGH, J. B. (1967). On the pattern of change in peripheral nerves produced by isoniazid intoxication in rats. *J. Neurol. Neurosurg. Psychiat.* **30,** 26.

CAVAZZANA, P. and BORSETTO, P. L. (1948). Recherches sur l'aspect microscopique des plexus nerveux intramuraux et sur les modifications morphologiques de leurs neurones dans les divers traits de l'intestin humain pendant la vie. *Acta Anat.* (*Basel*) **5,** 17.

CHAGAS, C. (1910). Aspecto clinico da nova entidade morbida produzid pelo. *Schizotrypanum Cruzi. Brasil med.* **24,** 263.

CHASE, M. R. and RANSON, S. W. (1914). The structure of the roots, trunk and branches of the vagus nerve. *J. comp. Neurol.* **24,** 31.

CHESTERMAN, J. T. (1946). Neurogenic ileus. *Brit. med. J.* **1,** 830.

CONNELL, A. M. (1969). The role of the pylorus in the aetiology of gastric ulcer. *Rend. Riunion. Rom. Gastroent.* **1,** 25.

COOKE, W. T., PEENEY, A. L. P. and HAWKINS, C. F. (1953). Symptoms, signs and diagnostic features of idiopathic steatorrhoea. *Quart. J. Med.* **22,** 59.

CORWIN, R. W. (1915). Megaduodenum. *Colo Med.* **12,** 138.

COUPLAND, R. E. and HOLMES, R. L. (1957). The use of cholinesterase techniques for the demonstration of peripheral nervous structures. *Quart. J. micr. Sci.* **98,** 327.

— (1958). Auerbach's plexus in the rabbit. *J. Anat.* **92,** 651.

CRAVER, W. L. (1957). Hypertrophic pyloric stenosis in adults. *Gastroenterology* **33** 914.

CREAMER, B., DONOGHUE, F. E. and CODE, C. F. (1968). Pattern of esophageal motility in diffuse spasm. *Gastroenterology* **54,** 775.

CREAMER, B., OLSEN, A. M. and CODE, C. F. (1957). The esophageal sphincters in achalasia of the cardia (cardiospasm). *Gastroenterology* **33,** 293.

CROSS, F. S. (1952). Pathologic changes in megaesophagus (esophageal dystonia). *Surgery* **31,** 647.

CRUVEILHIER, J. (1835). Rétrécissement du pylore. *Anat. path. Corps hum.* **1,** 4.

CRYMBLE, P. T. and WALMSLEY, T. (1933). 'Hypertrophy of the pylorus' in an adult. *Brit. J. Surg.* **20,** 602.

DALLA VALLIE, A. (1920). Ricerche istologiche su di un caso di megacolon congenito. *Pediatria* (*Napoli*) **28,** 740.

DELOYERS, L., DUPREZ, A. and BROMBART, M. (1959). Achalasia of the cardia experimentally produced in the cat by chemical destruction of Auerbach's plexus. *Acta chir. belg.* (Suppl.) **2,** 147.

DEREYMAEKER, A. (1943). Recherches expérimentales sur l'origine du système nerveux entérique chez l'embryon de poulet. *Arch. Biol.* (*Liège*) **54,** 359.

DERRICK, E. H. and GRAMBAUER, B. M. ST G. (1957). Megacolon in mice. *J. Path. Bact.* **73,** 569.

DE WOLFF, E. (1964). Étude clinique de 134 mongoliens. *Ann. paediat.* (*Basel*) **202,** Suppl. 47.

DODGE, J. A. (1967). ABO blood groups and infantile hypertrophic pyloric stenosis. *Brit. med. J.* **4,** 781.

DOGIEL, A. S. (1899). Ueber den Bau der Ganglien in den Geflechten des Darmes und der Gallenblase des Menschen und der Säugethiere. *Arch. Anat. physiol.* p. 130.

DONHOFFER, A. (1959). Feinere Lokalisation verschiedener Cholinesterasen der Nervösen Darmgeflechte. *Acta morph. Acad. Sci. hung.* **8,** 375.

DOUTHWAITE, A. H. and GOULDING, R. (1957). Action of senna. *Brit. med. J.* **2,** 1414.

DOWNES, W. A. (1917). Giant duodenum. *Ann. Surg.* **66,** 436.

DUDLEY, G. S. (1929). Duodenal dilatation. *Surg. Clin. N. Amer.* **9,** 667.

DUDLEY, H. A. F., SINCLAIR, I. S. R., MCLAREN, I. F., MCNAIR, J. J. and NEWSAM, J. E. (1958). Intestinal pseudo-obstruction. *J. roy. Coll. Edinb.* **3,** 206.

DUHAMEL, B. (1959). Exclusion du rectum avec abaissement rétrorectal et trans-anal du colon. Applications et premiers résultats d'une technique nouvelle. *Mem. Acad. Chir.* **85,** 192.

DU PLESSIS, D. J. (1966). Primary hypertrophic pyloric stenosis in the adult. *Brit. J. Surg.* **53,** 485.

DUPONT, J-R., JERVIS, H. R. and SPRINZ, H. (1965). A kinetic study of the myenteric neurones: size variations in the neurovegetative periphery with body weight and organ size. *Amer. J. Anat.* **116,** 335.

EARLAM, R. J., SCHLEGEL, J. F. and ELLIS, F. H., JR. (1967). Effect of ischaemia of lower esophagus and esophagogastric junction on canine esophageal motor function. *J. thorac. cardiovasc. Surg.* **54,** 822.

EDGEWORTH, F. H. (1892). On a large-fibred sensory supply of the thoracic and abdominal viscera. *J. Physiol.* (*Lond.*) **13,** 260.

EDWARDS, D. A. W. (1961). Physiological concepts of the pylorus. *Proc. roy. Soc. Med.* **54,** 930.

EDWARDS, H. C. (1936). Diverticulosis of the small intestine. *Ann. Surg.* **103,** 230.

EHRENPREIS, T. (1946). Megacolon in the newborn. *Acta chir. scand.* **94,** Suppl. 112.

ELLIOTT, T. R. and BARCLAY-SMITH, E. (1904). Antiperistalsis and other muscular. activities of the colon. *J. Physiol.* (*Lond.*) **31,** 272.

ELLIS, F. G., KAUNTZE, R., NIGHTINGALE, A. and TROUNCE, J. R. (1960). Further studies in achalasia of the cardia. *Quart. J. Med.* **29,** 305.

ELLIS, F. G., KAUNTZE, R. and TROUNCE, J. R. (1960). The innervation of the cardia and lower esophagus in man. *Brit. J. Surg.* **47,** 466.

EMANUEL, B., PADORR, M. P. and SWENSON, O. (1965). Mongolism associated with Hirschsprung's disease. *J. Pediat.* **66,** 437.

ERSKINE, J. M. (1963). Acquired megacolon, megaesophagus and megaduodenum with aperistalsis. *Amer. J. Gastroent.* **40,** 588.

ETZEL, E. (1937). Megaoesophagus and its neuropathology. *Guy's Hosp. Rep.* **87,** 158.

EVANS, D. H. L. and MURRAY, J. G. (1954*a*). Histological and functional studies on the fibre composition of the vagus nerve of the rabbit. *J. Anat.* **88,** 320.

— (1954*b*). Regeneration of non-medullated nerve fibres. *J. Anat.* **88,** 465.

FAIRBAIRN, J. W. (1958). Action of senna. *Brit. med. J.* **1,** 218.

FENWICK, T. (1953). Familial hypertrophic pyloric stenosis. *Brit. med. J.* **2,** 12.

FERGUSON, J. H. (1936). Effects of vagotomy on the gastric functions of monkeys. *Surg. Gynec. Obstet.* **62,** 689.

FERREIRA-SANTOS, R. and CARRIL, C. F. (1964). Acquired megacolon in Chagas' disease. *Dis. Colon Rect.* **7,** 353.

FINNEY, J. M. T. (1908). Congential idiopathic dilatation of the colon. *Surg. Gynec. Obstet.* **6,** 624.

FISCHER, H. (1909). Ueber funktionelle Anpassung am Fledermausmagan. *Arch. ges. physiol.* **129,** 113.

FISCHER, H. W. (1960). The big duodenum. *Amer. J. Roentgenol.* **83,** 861.

FOCK, G. and KOSTIA, J. (1963). Familial occurrence of Hirschsprung's disease. *Clin. Pediat.* (*Phila.*) **2,** 371.

FRIESEN, S. R., BOLEY, J. O. and MILLER, D. R. (1956). The myenteric plexus of the pylorus; its early normal development and its changes in hypertrophic pyloric stenosis. *Surgery* **39,** 21.

FRIESEN, S. R. and PEARSE, A. G. E. (1963). Pathogenesis of congenital pyloric stenosis: histochemical analyses of pyloric ganglion cells. *Surgery* **53,** 604.

FRORIEP, A. (1907). Ueber die Entwicklung und Bau des autonomen Nervensystems. *Med-Naturw. Arch.* **1,** 301.

GABELLA, G. (1967). Neurone number in the myenteric plexus in new-born and adult rats. *Experientia* **23,** 52.

GANDER, D. R. and DEVLIN, H. B. (1963). Ileus after amitriptyline. *Brit. med. J.* **1,** 1160.

GARRETT, J. R., HOWARD, E. R. and NIXON, H. H. (1969). Autonomic nerves in rectum and colon in Hirschsprung's disease. *Arch. Dis. Child.* **44,** 406.

GARRY, R. C. (1957). Innervation of abdominal viscera. *Brit. med. Bull.* **13,** 202.

GHORMLEY, R. K., HIGHTOWER, N. C., JR., CODE, C. F. and PRIESTLEY, J. T. (1954). Observations on intestinal motility through a paper-thin abdominal wall 14 years after removal of epithelioma; report of a case. *Proc. Mayo Clin.* **29,** 311.

GOLDBERG, I. H. (1965). Mode of action of antibiotics. (2) Drugs affecting nucleic acid and protein synthesis. *Amer. J. Med.* **39,** 722.

GORDON, H., TORRINGTON, M., LOUW, J. H., and CYWES, S. (1966). A genetical study of Hirschsprung's disease. Congenital intestinal agangliosis. *S. Afr. med. J.* **40,** 720.

GRABFIELD, G. P. (1937). New experiments on some old cathartics. *J. Pharmacol. exp. Ther.* **60,** 108.

GRAIVIER, L. and SIEBER, W. K. (1966). Hirschsprung's disease and mongolism. *Surgery* **60,** 458.

GREVING, R. (1952). Histologische Studien am Plexus myentericus des Magens. Ueber die Kontinuität von Ganglienzellen, das Terminalreticulum und das Synapse-Problem. *Acta neuroveg.* (*Wien*) **3,** 507.

GRONDAHL, J. W. and HANEY, H. F. (1940). Attempt to produce experimental cardiospasm in dogs. *Proc. Soc. exp. Biol. Med.* **44,** 126.

GUNN, M. (1959). Cell types in the myenteric plexus of the cat. *J. comp. Neurol.* **111,** 83.

— (1968). Histological and histochemical observations on the myenteric and submucous plexuses of mammals. *J. Anat.* **102,** 223.

HARRIS, L. D., ASHWORTH, W. D. and INGELFINGER, F. J. (1960). Esophageal aperistalsis and achalasia produced in dogs by prolonged cholinesterase inhibition. *J. clin. Invest.* **39,** 1744.

HAWKINS, D. B. (1958). Action of senna. *Brit. med. J.* **1,** 281.

HERBST, C. (1934). Mikroskopische Untersuchungen der intramuralen Magennerven beim Pylospasmus. *Z. Kinderheilk.* **56,** 122.

HERTZ (HURST), A. F. and NEWTON, A. (1913). The normal movements of the colon in man. *J. Physiol.* (*Lond.*) **47,** 57.

HERTZ, R., LIPSETT, M. B. and MOY, R. H. (1960). Effect of vincaleukoblastine on metastatic choriocarcinoma and related trophoblastic tumors in women. *Cancer Res.* **20,** 1050.

HEYROWSKY, H. (1913). Casuistik und Therapie der idiopathischen Dilatation der Speiseöhre. Oesophagogastroanastomose. *Arch. klin. Chir.* **100,** 703.

HIEBERT, B. W. and FARRIS, J. M. (1966). Hypertrophic pyloric stenosis in the adult. Review of 22 cases. *Amer. Surg.* **32,** 712.

HIGGS, B., KERR, F. W. L. and ELLIS, F. H., JR. (1965). The experimental production of esophageal achalasia by electrolytic lesions in the medulla. *J. thorac. cardiovasc. Surg.* **50,** 613.

HILL, C. J. (1927). A contribution to our knowledge of the enteric plexuses. *Phil. Trans. B* **215,** 355.

HILLARP, N. A. (1959). The construction and functional organization of the autonomic innervation apparatus. *Acta physiol. scand.* **46,** Suppl. 157.

HIRSCHSPRUNG, H. (1888*a*). Stuhlträgheit Neugeborer in Folge von Dilatation und Hypertrophie des Colons. *Jb. Kinderheilk.* **27,** 1.

— (1888*b*). Fälle von angeborener pylorusstenose, beobachtet bei saüglingen. *Jb. Kinderheilk.* **28,** 61.

HOFFMAN, H. H. (1956). Fibre components of the vagus nerve in man. *Anat. Rec.* **124,** 306.

HOFMEISTER, F. and SCHÜTZ, E. (1886). Ueber die automatischen Bewegungen des Magen. *Arch. exp. Path. Pharmakol.* **20,** 1.

HOLT, S. J. (1959). Factors governing the validity of staining methods for enzymes and their bearing on the Gomori acid phosphatase technique. *Exp. Cell Res.* Suppl. **7,** 1.

HOLZKNECHT, C. (1909). Die normale Peristaltik des Kolon. *Münch. med. Wschr.* **56,** 2401.

HONJIN, R. (1951). Studies on the nerve endings in the small intestine. *Cytol. Neurol. Stud. Kanazawa* **9,** 1.

HONJIN, R., IZUMI, S. and OSUGI, H. (1959). The distribution and morphology of argentophile and argentophobe nerve cells in the myenteric plexus of the digestive tube of the mouse: a quantitative study. *J. comp. Neurol.* **111,** 291.

HORTON, B. T. (1928). Pyloric musculature with special reference to pyloric block. *Arch. Surg.* **22,** 438.

HOUGHTON, B. J. and PEARS, M. A. (1958). Chronic potassium depletion due to purgation with cascara. *Brit. med. J.* **1,** 1328.

HUKUHARA, T., KOTANI, S. and SATO, G. (1961). Effects of destruction of intramural ganglion cells on colon motility: possible genesis of congenital megacolon. *Jap. J. Physiol.* **11,** 635.

HUKUHARA, T., SUMI, T. and KOTANI, S. (1961). The role of the ganglion cells in the small intestine taken in the intestinal intrinsic reflex. *Jap. J. Physiol.* **11,** 281.

HUNTER, R. H. (1933). A case of megaduodenum with multiple anomalies of the ileum. *Arch. Dis. Child.* **8,** 155.

HUNTER, R., EARL, C. J. and THORNICROFT, S. (1964). An apparently irreversible syndrome of abnormal movements following phenothiazine medication. *Proc. roy. Soc. Med.* **57,** 758.

HURST, A. F. (1934). Some disorders of the esophagus. *J. Amer. med. Ass.* **102,** 582.

HURST, A. F. and RAKE, G. W. (1930). Achalasia of the cardia. *Quart. J. Med.* **23,** 491.

INGELFINGER, F. J. (1943). The diagnosis of sprue in non-tropical areas. *New Engl. J. Med.* **228,** 180.

IORDANSKAIA, N. I. (1962). Functional disorders of the vagus nerves in cardiospasm. *Vestn. Khir.* **88,** 24.

IRWIN, D. A. (1931). The anatomy of Auerbach's plexus. *Amer. J. Anat.* **49,** 141.

JABONERO, V. (1951). Organizacion anatomica y fisiologica del sistema neurovegetativo periferico. *Acta argent. fisiol. y fisiopath.* **1,** 579.

JACKSON, R. G. (1949). Anatomy of the vagus nerves in the region of the lower esophagus and the stomach. *Anat. Rec.* **103,** 1.

JACOBOWITZ, D. (1965). Histochemical studies of the autonomic innervation of the gut. *J. Pharmacol. exp. Ther.* **149,** 358.

JENNINGS, P. J. (1967). Megarectum and megacolon in adolescents and young adults. *Proc. roy. Soc. Med.* **60,** 805.

JEWETT, C. H. (1928). Chronic duodenal ileus. *J. Amer. med. Ass.* **91,** 91.

JOHNSON, S. E. (1925). Experimental degeneration of the extrinsic nerves of the small intestine in relation to the structure of the myenteric plexus. *J. comp. Neurol.* **38,** 299.

JOHNSTON, I. D. A. and GIBSON, J. B. (1959). Megacolon and volvulus in psychotics. *Brit. J. Surg.* **47,** 394.

JONES, D. S. (1942). The origin of the vagi and the parasympathetic ganglion cells of the viscera of the chick. *Anat. Rec.* **82,** 185.

JONES, F. A. (1967). Cathartic colon. *Proc. roy. Soc. Med.* **60,** 503.

KAY, E. B. (1951). Observations as to the etiology and treatment of achalasia of the esophagus. *J. thorac. Surg.* **22,** 254.

KEELER, R., RICHARDSON, H. and WATSON, A. J. (1966). Enteromegaly and steatorrhoea in the rat following intraperitoneal quinacrine (atabrine). *Lab. Invest.* **15,** 1253.

KEYNES, W. M. (1965). Simple and complicated hypertrophic stenosis in the adult. *Gut* **6,** 240.

KIMURA, K. (1929). The nature of idiopathic esophagus dilatation. *Jap. J. Gastroent.* **1,** 199.

KLINGHARDT, G. W. (1954). Experimentelle Nervenfaserschädigungen durch Isonicotinsäurehydrazid und ihre Bedeutung für die Klinik. *Verh. dtsch. Ges. inn. Med.* **60,** 764.

KNIGHT, C. D. (1961). Hypertrophic pyloric stenosis in the adult. *Ann. Surg.* **153,** 899.

KNIGHT, G. C. (1934). The innervation of the oesophagus and cardiac sphincter. *J. Physiol.* (*Lond.*) **81,** 6p.

KÖBERLE, F. (1957). Ueber Enteromegalie. *Zbl. allg. Path. path. Anat.* **96,** 244.

— (1963). Enteromegaly and cardiomegaly in Chagas' disease. *Gut* **4,** 399.

KOELLE, G. B. (1955). The histochemical identification of acetyl cholinesterase in cholinergic, adrenergic and sensory neurons. *J. Pharmacol. exp. Ther.* **114,** 167.

KOELLE, G. B. and FRIEDENWALD, J. S. (1949). A histochemical method for localizing cholinesterase activity. *Proc. Soc. exp. Biol. Med.* **70,** 617.

KOELLE, G. B. and GILMAN, A. (1946). The chronic toxicity of di-isopropyl fluorophosphate (DFP) in dogs, monkeys and rats. *J. Pharmacol. exp. Ther.* **87,** 435.

KOHN, A. (1907). Ueber die Entwicklung des sympathischen Nervensystems der Säugetiere. *Arch. mikrosk. Anat.* **70,** 266.

KÖLLIKER, A. (1896). *Lehrbuch der Gewebelehre*, Bd. 2. Leipzig.

KRAAS, E. (1933). Beitrag zur Ätiologie und Klinik der chronischen Duodenalstenose und des Megaduodenums. *Beitr. klin. Chir.* **157,** 489.

KRAMER, P. and INGELFINGER, F. J. (1949). Motility of the human esophagus in control subjects and in patients with esophageal disorders. *Amer. J. Med.* **7,** 168.

KRAMER, P., INGELFINGER, F. J. and ATKINSON, M. (1956). The motility and pharmacology of the esophagus in cardiospasm. *Int. Congr. Gastroent.* **5,** 174.

KRAUS, F. (1902). Krankheiten des Oesophagus. *Nothnagels Handbuch.* Wien: Alfred Hölder.

KUNTZ, A. (1910). The development of the sympathetic nervous system in mammals. *J. comp. Neurol.* **20,** 211.

— (1911). The evolution of the sympathetic nervous system in vertebrates. *J. comp. Neurol.* **21,** 215.

— (1920). The development of the sympathetic nervous system in man. *J. comp. Neurol.* **32,** 173.
— (1922). On the occurrence of reflex arcs in the myenteric and submucous plexuses. *Anat. Rec.* **24,** 193.
— (1952). Origin and early development of the pelvic neural plexuses. *J. comp. Neurol.* **96,** 345.

LANE, P. W. (1966). Association of megacolon with two recessive spotting genes in the mouse. *J. Hered.* **57,** 29.
LANGLEY, J. N. (1891). The innervation of the pelvic viscera. *J. Physiol.* (*Lond.*) **12,** 23.
— (1922). Connexions of the enteric nerve cells. *J. Physiol.* (*Lond.*) **56,** 39.
LANGLEY, J. N. and ANDERSON, H. K. (1894). The constituents of the hypogastric nerves. *J. Physiol.* (*Lond.*) **17,** 177.
— (1895). On the innervation of the pelvic and adjoining viscera. (1) The lower portion of the intestine. *J. Physiol.* (*Lond.*) **18,** 67.
LANNON, J. and WELLER, E. (1947). The parasympathetic supply of the distal colon. *Brit. J. Surg.* **34,** 373.
LARANJA, F. S., DIAS, E., NORBREGA, G. and MIRANDA, A. (1956). Chagas' disease. A clinical, epidemiologic and pathologic study. *Circulation* **14,** 1035.
LA VILLA, S. (1897). Estructura de los ganglios intestinales. *Rev. trimest. Microgr. Madrid* **11,** 187.
LAWRENTJEW, B. J. (1925). Ueber die nervose Natur und das Vorkommen der sogenannten 'interstitial Zellen' (Cajal, Dogiel) in der glatten Muskulatur. *Proc. med. Akad. Wet.* **28,** 977.
— (1931). Zur Lehre von der Cytoarchitektonik des peripherischen autonomen Nervensystems. (1) Die Cytoarchitektonik der Ganglien des Verdauungskanals beim Hunde. *Z. mikr.-anat. Forsch.* **23,** 527.
LEAMING, D. B. and CAUNA, N. (1961). A qualitative and quantitative study of the myenteric plexus of the small intestine of the cat. *J. Anat.* **95,** 160.
LEARMONTH, J. R. and MARKOWITZ, J. (1930). Studies on the innervation of the large bowel. (2) The influence of the lumbar colonic nerves on the distal part of the colon. *Amer. J. Physiol.* **94,** 501.
LEHMANN, G. (1945). Gastric cardiospasm in the dog. *Amer. J. Physiol.* **143,** 163.
LENDRUM, F. C. (1937). Anatomic features of the cardiac orifice of the stomach. *Arch. intern. Med.* **59,** 474.
LERCHE, W. (1950). *The Esophagus and Pharynx in Action. A Study of Structure in Relation to Function.* Springfield, Illinois: Thomas.
LERMAN, L. S. (1961). Structural considerations in the interactions of DNA and acridines. *J. molec. Biol.* **3,** 18.
LEVIN, A. (1923). Duodenal dilatation. *New Orleans med. Surg. J.* **4, 76,** 178
LI, P. L. (1939). The intramural nervous system of the small intestine with special reference to the innervation of the inner subdivision of its circular muscle. *J. anat.* **74,** 348.
LOEPER, M. and FORESTIER, J. (1921). Les lésions nerveuses du pneumogastrique et le cardiospasme récurrent dans le cancer de l'estomac. *Arch. Mal. Appar. dig.* **11,** 307.
LONG, D. M., NICE, C. M., JR., THAL, A. P. and TRUEX, R. C. (1958). The experimental production of cardiospasm in dogs. *Surg. Forum* **9,** 408.
LUMSDEN, K. and TRUELOVE, S. C. (1958). Primary hypertrophic pyloric stenosis in the adult. *Brit. J. Radiol.* **31,** 261.

MCCLELLAND, H. A., LEWIS, M. J. and NAISH, J. M. (1962). Idiopathic steatorrhoea with intestinal pseudo-obstruction. *Gut* **3,** 142.

MCCREA, E. D'A. (1924). The abdominal distribution of the vagus. *J. Anat.* **59,** 18

MCCREA, E. D'A. and MCSWINEY, B. A. (1928). The effect on the stomach of stimulation of the peripheral end of the splanchnic nerve. *Quart. J. exp. Physiol.* **18,** 301.

MACMAHON, B. and MCKEOWN, T. (1955). Infantile hypertrophic pyloric stenosis. Data on 81 pairs of twins. *Acta Genet. med.* (*Roma*) **4,** 320.

MALL, F. (1896). A study of the intestinal contraction. *Johns Hopk. Hosp. Rep.* **1,** 37.

MANN, C. V. and SHORTER, R. G. (1964). Structure of the canine esophagus and its sphincters. *J. surg. Res.* **4,** 160.

MARCUS, H. (1909). Ueber den Sympathicus. *Jber. ges. Morph. Physiol. Münch.* **25,** 119.

MARKS, B. H., SAMORAJSKI, T. and WEBSTER, E. J. (1962). Radioautographic localization of norepinephrine H3 in the tissues of mice. *J. Pharmacol. exp. Ther.* **138,** 376.

MARTINDALE (1967). *Extra Pharmacopoeia* (edited by Todd, R. G.). 25th edition.

MASLENNIKOVA, L. D. (1962). On the relation between the motor function of the intestine and the gradient of its nervous elements. *Bull. exp. Biol. Med.* **52,** 972.

MEISSNER, G. (1857). Ueber die Nerven der Darmwand. *Z. ration. Med.* **8,** 364.

MELCHIOR, E. (1924). Beiträge zur chirurgischen duodenalpathologie das Megaduodenum. *Arch. klin. Chir.* **128**, 1.

MELTZER, S. J. and AUER, J. (1906). Vagus reflexes upon oesophagus and cardia. *Brit. med. J.* **2,** 1806.

METRAKOS, J. D. (1953). Congenital hypertrophic pyloric stenosis in twins. *Arch. Dis. Child.* **28,** 351.

MEYLING, H. A. (1953). Structure and significance of the perpheral extension of the autonomic nervous system. *J. comp. Neurol.* **99,** 495.

MICHAIL, S. and KARAMANDLIDIS, A. (1967). Morphologie du plexus myenterique d'Auerbach de l'intestin grêle du chien. *Acta Anat.* (*Basel*) **67,** 424.

MIHICH, E. and NICHOL, C. A. (1959). The effect of pyridoxine deficiency on mouse sarcoma 180. *Cancer Res.* **19,** 279.

MISIEWICZ, J. J., WALLER, S. L., ANTHONY, P. P. and GUMMER, J. W. P. (1969). Achalasia of the cardia. Pharmacology and histophathology of isolated cardiac sphincteric muscle from patients with and without achalasia. *Quart. J. Med.* **38,** 17.

MITCHELL, G. A. G. (1935). The innervation of the distal colon. *Edinb. med. J.* **42,** 11.

— (1940). A macroscopic study of the nerve supply of the stomach. *J. Anat.* **75,** 50.

MODERN, F. S. and THIENES, C. H. (1936). Vagal and sympathetic endings in the rabbit intestine. *Science* **83,** 522.

MORRISON, A. R. and HABEL, R. E. (1964). A quantitative study of the distribution of vagal nerve endings in the myenteric plexus of the ruminant stomach. *J. comp. Neurol.* **122,** 297.

MOSHER, H. P. and MCGREGOR, G. W. (1928). A study of the lower end of the esophagus. *Ann. Otol.* **37,** 12.

MÜLLER, L. R. (1911). Die Darminnervation. *Dtsch. Arch. klin. Med.* **105,** 1.

MURAKAMI, T. (1934). Neurohistologische Untersuchungen über das Ostium iliocaecocolicum des Hundes. *Jap. J. med. Sci. Anat.* **4,** 417.

NAISH, J. M., CAPPER, W. M. and BROWN, N. J. (1960). Intestinal pseudo-obstruction with steatorrhoea. *Gut.* **1,** 62.

NELL, W. (1932). Ueber das Megaduodenum. *Zbl. Chir.* **59,** 2997.

NEMIR, P. and HAWTHORNE, H. R. (1954). Physiologic basis for utilization of esophago-cardiomyotomy in the treatment of achalasia. *J. thorac. Surg.* **28,** 247.

NIEMI, M., KOUVALAINEN, K. and HJELT, L. (1961). Cholinesterases and monoamine oxidase in congenital megacolon. *J. Path. Bact.* **82,** 363.

NIXON, H. H. (1964). Hirschsprung's disease. *Arch. Dis. Child.* **39,** 109.

NORBERG, K. A. (1964). Adrenergic innervation of the intestinal wall studied by fluorescence microscopy. *Int. J. Neuropharmacol.* **3,** 379.

NORTH, J. P. and JOHNSON, J. H., JR. (1950). Pyloric hypertrophy in the adult. *Ann. Surg.* **131,** 316.

OKADA, T. (1940). Ueber den Mechanismus der Sennaabführung. *Tohoku J. exp. Med.* **38,** 33.

OKAMOTO, E., IWASAKI, T., UEDA, T. and TAKEDA, Y. (1964). Pathogenesis of cardiospasm, clincial and experimental studies. *Med. J. Osaka Univ.* **14,** 245.

OKAMOTO, E., IWASAKI, T. and KAKUTANI, T. (1967). Selective destruction of the myenteric plexus: its relation to Hirschsprung's disease, achalasia of the esophagus and hypertrophic pyloric stenosis. *J. pediat. Surg.* **2,** 444.

OKAMOTO, E., KAKUTANI, T., IWASAKI, T., NAMBA, M. and UEDA, T. (1964). Morphological studies on the myenteric plexus of the colon in chronic ulcerative colitis. A preliminary report. *Med. J. Osaka Univ.* **15,** 85.

OKAMOTO, E. and UEDA, T. (1967). Embryogenesis of intramural ganglia of the gut and its relation to Hirschsprung's disease. *J. pediat. Surg.* **2,** 437.

OKUMURA, M. and NETO, A. C. (1961). Producao experimental de 'megas' en animais inoculados com *Trypanosoma cruzi*. *Rev. Hosp. Clín. Fac. Med. S. Paulo* **16,** 338.

ÖNODI, A. D. (1886). Ueber die Entwickelung des sympathischen Nervensystems. *Arch. mikrosk. Anat.* **26,** 61.

ORF, G. (1965). Das vegetative Nervensystem bei Colitis ulcerosa. *Dtsch. Z. Nervenheilk.* **187,** 837.

OSLER, W. (1881). Notes on intestinal diverticula. *Ann. anat. Surg.* **2,** 202.

PASSARGE, E. (1967). The genetics of Hirschsprung's disease. Evidence for heterogeneous etiology and a study of 63 families. *New Engl. J. Med.* **276,** 138.

PETREN, G. (1936). Ein Fall von Megaduodenum nebst einigen Bemerkungen über die Genese und Klinik der chronischen Duodenaldilatation. *Acta chir. scand.* **77,** 307.

PHILLIPS, J. H. C. (1952). Jejunal diverticulosis, some clinical aspects. *Brit. J. Surg.* **40,** 350.

PIERANDOZZI, J. S. and RITTER, J. H. (1966). Transient achalasia. A complication of vagotomy. *Amer. J. Surg.* **111,** 356.

QUIGLEY, J. P. and LOUCKES, H. (1952). Pyloric sphincter activity in normal dog. *Fed. Proc.* **11,** 125.

RAIA, A. (1943). *Acalasia do piloro.* Tese. S. Paulo.

RAIA, A., ACQUARONI, D. and NETTO, A. C. (1961). Pathogenesis and treatment of acquired megaduodenum. *Amer. J. dig. Dis.* **6,** 757.

RAIA, A., CURTI, P., ALMEIDA, A. and FRY, W. (1956). The pathogenesis of hypertrophic stenosis of the pylorus in the newborn and the adult. *Surg. Gynec. Obstet.* **102,** 705.

RAKE, G. W. (1926). A case of annular muscular hypertrophy of the oesophagus (achalasia of the cardia without oesophageal dilatation). *Guy's Hosp. Rep.* **76,** 145.

— (1927). On the pathology of achalasia of the cardia. *Guy's Hosp. Rep.* **77,** 141.

RASH, R. M. and THOMAS, M. D. (1962). The intrinsic innervation of the gastro-oesophageal and pyloro-duodenal junctions. *J. Anat.* **96,** 389.

REID, P. E., IVY, A. C. and QUIGLEY, J. P. (1934). Spiral propulsion of a bolus in the intestine. *Amer. J. Physiol.* **109,** 483.

REMAK, R. (1847). *Ueber ein selbständiges Darmnervensystem.* Berlin.

REYES, F. A., JR. and FRIESEN, S. R. (1967). Review of the neuromuscular abnormalities in achalasia of the oesophagus, congenital pyloric stenosis and congenital aganglionic megacolon. *Rev. Surg.* (*Phila.*) **24,** 153.

RICHARDSON, K. C. (1958). Electronmicroscopic observations on Auerbach's plexus in the rabbit, with special reference to the problem of smooth muscle innervation. *Amer. J. Anat.* **103,** 99.

— (1960). Studies on the structure of autonomic nerves in the small intestine, correlating the silver-impregnated image in light microscopy with the permanganate-fixed ultrastructure in electron microscopy. *J. Anat.* **94,** 457.

RINTOUL, J. R. (1959). The comparative morphology of the enteric neurones. *J. Anat.* **93,** 583.

RINTOUL, J. R. and KIRKMAN, N. F. (1961). The myenteric plexus in infantile hypertrophic pyloric stenosis. *Arch. Dis. Child.* **36,** 474.

ROBERTS, P. A. L. (1959). Pathology of infantile hypertrophic pyloric stenosis. *Proc. roy. Soc. Med.* **52,** 1022.

ROBERTSON, H. E. and KERNOHAN, J. W. (1938). The myenteric plexus in congenital megacolon. *Proc. Mayo Clin.* **13,** 123.

RUNSTRÖM, G. (1939). On the roentgen-anatomical appearance of congenital pyloric stenosis during and after the manifest stage of the disease. *Acta paediat.* **26,** 383.

SAUER, M. E. and RUMBLE, C. T. (1946). The number of nerve cells in the myenteric and submucous plexuses of the small intestine of the cat. *Anat. Rec.* **96,** 373.

SCHMIDT, C. A. (1933). Distribution of vagus and sacral nerves to the large intestine. *Proc. Soc. exp. Biol. Med.* **30,** 739.

SCHMIDT, J. E. (1909). Ueber Hirschsprung'sche Krankheit insbesondere ihre chirurgische Behandlung. *Beitr. klin. Chir.* **61,** 682.

SCHOCHET, S. S., JR., LAMPERT, P. W. and EARLE, K. M. (1968). Neuronal changes induced by intrathecal vincristine sulphate. *J. Neuropath. exp. Neurol.* **27,** 645.

SCHOFIELD, G. C. (1957). An experimental study of the extrinsic nerve supply of the alimentary tract in the rat. *J. Anat.* **91,** 593.

— (1960). Experimental studies of the innervation of the mucous membrane of the gut. *Brain* **83,** 490.

— (1962). Experimental studies on the myenteric plexus in mammals. *J. comp. Neurol.* **119,** 159.

SCHWARTZ, W. B. and RELMAN, A. S. (1953). Metabolic and renal studies in chronic potassium depletion resulting from overuse of laxatives. *J. clin. Invest.* **32,** 258.

SHELANSKI, M. L. and WISNIEWSKI, H. (1969). Neurofibrillary degeneration induced by vincristine therapy. *Arch. Neurol.* (*Chic.*) **20,** 199.

SIEGMUND, H. (1935). Anatomisch nachgewiesene Folgen von Tonus und Motilitatsstörungen des Verdauundskanals bei Enzephalitikern die mit Atropin behandelt wurden. *Münch. med. Wschr.* **82,** 453.

SMITH, B. (1967*a*). Myenteric plexus in Hirschsprung's disease. *Gut* **8,** 308.

— (1967*b*). The myenteric plexus in Chagas' disease. *J. Path. Bact.* **94,** 462.

— (1967*c*). The myenteric plexus in drug-induced neuropathy. *J. Neurol. Neurosurg. Psychiat.* **30,** 506.

— (1968). Effect of irritant purgatives on the myenteric plexus in man and the mouse. *Gut,* **9,** 139.

— (1969). Damage to the intrinsic cardiac neurones by rubidomycin (daunorubicin). *Brit. Heart J.* **31,** 607.

SPOERRI, R. (1949). Histological studies on nerve elements and their endings at epithelial cells of the gastric mucosa. *J. comp. Neurol.* **90,** 151.

STOERK, H. C. and EISEN, H. N. (1946). Suppression of circulating antibodies in pyridoxin deficiency. *Proc. Soc. exp. Biol. Med.* **62,** 88.

STÖHR, P., JR. (1930). Mikroskopische Studien zur Innervation des Magendarmkanales. *Z. Zellforsch.* **12,** 66.

— (1949). Mikroskopische Studien zur Innervation des Magendarmkanales. V. *Z. Zellforsch.* **34,** 1.

STORSTEEN, K. A., KERNOHAN, K. W. and BARGEN, J. A. (1953). The myenteric plexus in chronic ulcerative colitis. *Surg. Gynec. Obstet.* **97,** 335.

STRAUB, W. and TRIENDL, E. (1937). Theorie der Abfuhrwirkung der Folia Sennae und ihre wirksamen Inhaltsstoffe. *Arch. exp. Path. Pharmakol.* **185,** 1.

SVENSON, O. and BILL, A. H. (1948). Resection of rectum and rectosigmoid with preservation of the sphincter for benigh spastic lesions producing megacolon. *Surgery* **24,** 212.

SYMONDS, C. P. (1930). quoted by Hurst and Rake.

TANNER, N. C. (1964). The surgical treatment of peptic ulcer. *Brit. J. Surg.* **51,** 5.

TAXI, J. (1961). Sur l'innervation des fibres musculaires lisses de l'intestin de souris. *C. R. Acad. Sci. (Paris)* **252,** 331.

TELFORD, E. D. and STOPFORD, J. S. B. (1934). The autonomic nerve supply of the distal colon. *Brit. med. J.* **1,** 572.

TELLO, J. F. (1924). La précocité embryonnaire du plexus d'Auerbach et ses différences dans les intestins antérieur et postérieur. *Trab. lab. Invest. Biol. Univ. Madr.* **22,** 317.

TEMPLETON, F. E. (1948). Movements of the esophagus in the presence of cardiospasm and other esophageal diseases. *Gastroenterology* **10,** 96.

TEMPLETON, R. D. and LAWSON, H. (1932). Studies in the motor activity of the large intestine. IV. *Amer. J. Physiol.* **101,** 511.

THOMAS, G. A. and TROUNCE, J. R. (1960). The effect of neuromuscular and ganglion blockade on the function of the guinea-pig oesophagus. *Guy's Hosp. Rep.* **109,** 21.

THOMAS, J. E. (1929). A further study of the nervous control of the pyloric sphincter. *Amer. J. Physiol.* **88,** 498.

— (1931). The mechanism of gastric evacuation. *J. Amer. med. Ass.* **97,** 1663.

— (1957). Mechanics and regulation of gastric emptying. *Physiol. Rev.* **37,** 453.

THOMAS, J. E. and KUNTZ, A. (1926). A study of gastro-intestinal motility in relation to the enteric nervous system. *Amer. J. Physiol.* **76,** 606.

THOMAS, J. E. and WHEELON, H. (1922). The nervous control of the pyloric sphincter. *J. Lab. clin. Med.* **7,** 375.

THOMPSON, J. (1950). Neuromuscular incoordination at the cardia in the newborn. *Arch. Dis. Child.* **25,** 52.

THOMSON, J. (1921). Observations on congenital hypertrophy of the pylorus. *Edinb. med. J.* **26,** 1.

TIFFIN, M. E., CHANDLER, L. R. and FABER, H. K. (1940). Localised absence of the ganglion cells of the myenteric plexus in congenital megacolon. *Amer. J. Dis. Child.* **59,** 1071.

TITTEL, K. (1901). Ueber eine angeborene Missbildung des Dickdarmes. *Wien. klin. Wschr.* **14,** 903.

TOBIN, W. E. and SANDLER, G. (1966). Depression of muscle spindle function with vincristine. *Nature (Lond.)* **212,** 90.

TRAVELL, J. (1954). Pharmacology of stimulant laxatives. *Ann. N.Y. Acad. Sci.* **58,** 416.

TRENDELENBURG, P. (1917). Physiologische und pharmakologische Versuche über die Dünndarmperistaltik. *Arch. exp. Path. Pharmakol.* **81,** 55.

TROUNCE, J. R., DEUCHAR, D. C., KAUNTZE, R. and THOMAS, G. A. (1957). Studies in achalasia of the cardia. *Quart. J. Med.* **26,** 433.

TROUNCE, J. R. and NIGHTINGALE, A. (1960). Studies in Hirschsprung's disease. *Arch. Dis. Child.* **35,** 373.

TRUELOVE, S. C. (1966). Movements of the large intestine. *Physiol. Rev.* **46,** 457.

VAN CAMPENHOUT, E. (1932). Further experiments on the origin of the enteric nervous system in the chick. *Physiol. Zool.* **5,** 333.

VICTOR, M. and ADAMS, R. D. (1956). Symposium on role of some newer vitamins in human metabolism and nutrition. The neuropathology of experimental vitamin B6 deficiency in monkeys. *Amer. J. clin. Nutr.* **4,** 346.

VIEIRA, C. B., DE GODOY, R. A. and CARRIL, C. F. (1964). Hypersensitivity of the large intestine to cholinergic agents in patients with Chagas' disease and megacolon. *Rev. bras. Gastroent.* **16,** 41.

WADDELL, M. C. (1929). Anatomical evidence for existence of enteric reflex arcs following degeneration of extrinsic nerves. *Proc. Soc. exp. Biol. Med.* **26,** 867.

WALLGREN, A. (1946). Preclinical stage of infantile hypertrophic pyloric stenosis. *Amer. J. Dis. Child.* **72,** 371.

WEISS, W. (1938). Zur ätiologie des Megaduodenums. *Dtsch. Z. Chir.* **251,** 317.

WELCH, P. B. and PLANT, O. H. (1926). A graphic study of muscular activity of the colon with special reference to its response to feeding. *Amer. J. med. Sci.* **172,** 261.

WHITEHOUSE, F. R. and KERNOHAN, J. W. (1948). Myenteric plexus in congenital megacolon. *Arch. intern. Med.* **82,** 75.

WILLIAMS, I. (1962). Closure of the pylorus. *Brit. J. Radiol.* **35,** 653.

WISNIEWSKI, H., SHELANSKI, M. L. and TERRY, R. D. (1968). Effects of mitotic spindle inhibitors on neurotubules and neurofilaments of anterior horn cells. *J. cell Biol.* **38,** 224.

WOOD, E. C. and SMELLIE, J. M. (1951). Congenital hypertrophic pyloric stenosis. *Lancet* **ii,** 3.

WOODBURNE, R. T. (1956). The sacral parasympathetic innervation of the colon. *Anat. Rec.* **124,** 67.

WOOLAM, G. L., MAHER, F. T. and ELLIS, F. H., JR. (1967). Vagal nerve function in achalasia of the esophagus. *Surg. Forum* **18,** 362.

WOOLLARD, H. H. (1935). The peripheral sympathetic nervous system. *Brit. J. Surg.* **23,** 425.

WOO-MING, M. (1961). Familial relationship between adult and infantile hypertrophic pyloric stenosis. *Brit. med. J.* **1,** 476.

WORLD HEALTH ORGANISATION (1960). Chagas' disease. *Wld Hlth Org. techn. Rep. Ser.* p. 202.

WRIGHT, P. G. and SHEPHERD, J. J. (1965). Response to drugs of isolated human colonic muscle from a case of Hirschsprung's disease. *Lancet* **ii,** 1161.

YNTEMA, C. L. and HAMMOND, W. S. (1947). The development of the autonomic nervous system. *Biol. Rev.* **22,** 344.

— (1953). Experiments on the sacral parasympathetic nerves and ganglia of the chick embryo. *Anat. Rec.* **115,** 382.

— (1954). The origin of intrinsic ganglia of trunk viscera from vagal neural crest in the chick embryo. *J. comp. Neurol.* **101,** 515.

ZBINDEN, G. and STÜDER, A. (1955). Experimenteller Beitrag zur Frage der Isoniazid-neuritis und ihrer Beeinflussung durch Pyridoxin. *Z. Tuberk.* **107,** 97.

ZIMMERMAN, G. R. (1962). Megacolon from large doses of chlorpromazine. *Arch. Path.* **74,** 47.
ZUELZER, W. W. and WILSON, J. L. (1948). Functional intestinal obstruction on a congenital neurogenic basis in infancy. *Amer. J. Dis. Child.* **75,** 40.

Index